French Toast
for Breakfast

Declaring
Peace with
Emotional Eating

Mary Anne Cohen

gürze books

FRENCH TOAST FOR BREAKFAST
Declaring Peace with Emotional Eating

©1995 by Mary Anne Cohen

Gürze Books
P.O. Box 2238
Carlsbad, CA 92018
(619) 434-7533

Cover design by Abacus Graphics, Oceanside, CA
Cover illustration by George Dimichina

Library of Congress Cataloging-in-Publication Data
French toast for breakfast: declaring peace with emotional eating / by Mary Anne Cohen
   p. cm.
   ISBN 0-936077-22-0
   1. Food habits—Psychological aspects. 2. Eating disorders. 3. Self-help techniques. I. Title
RC552.C65   1995   95-75215
616.85'26—dc20   CIP

NOTE:
The author and publisher of this book intend for this publication to provide accurate information. It is sold with the understanding that it is meant to complement, not substitute for, professional medical and/or psychological services.

4 6 8 0 9 7 5 3

*To Michael Scanlon
father of this book
whose vitality, love, and humor
are vitamins to my soul*

Contents

Acknowledgements

I would like to express my deep gratitude to Aaron, who cherished the little girl inside me and helped her grow; to my mother, Lily Lifshutz, whose imagination, humor, and curiosity about life are the fabric of who I am; to my father, Leon Lifshutz, whose gift of story-telling inspired me to want to write my own book.

I also appreciate the support provided me by the women in my life whose love and encouragement have been beyond compare. Thanks to Sharon Franz, Joan Furedi, Esther Garcia, Joanne Gerr, Martha Gunzburg, Celene Krauss, Lynda Pizer, Andrea Schneer, Mary Ellen Tyrmand, and Claire Zander. A special thanks to Lindsey Hall for all her editorial guidance along the way.

Finally, I would like to acknowledge the loving memory of my grandmothers, Jenny Hershman and Pauline Lifshutz.

All names and identifying characteristics of individuals mentioned in this book have been changed in order to protect their privacy.

Declaring Peace is an Inside Job

Now that my ladder is gone,
I must lie down where all ladders start,
In the foul rag and bones shop of the heart.
—W.B. Yeats

A colleague of mine, a psychologist, was describing to me how he uses hypnotherapy to help patients resolve their bingeing problems. "This is what I do," he began. "I tell my patients to imagine their favorite binge food. Very often it is chocolate. Then I lead them into a hypnotic trance, and while they are in the trance I advise them as follows: 'If you ever put a piece of chocolate in your mouth again, little eggs in that chocolate will crack open, and tiny worms will come out. These worms will crawl all over your mouth and into your stomach, ripping it apart. You will never be interested in eating chocolate again.' "

As he sat back, pleased at his inventiveness, I realized we were worlds apart in our thinking about how to help people heal from eating problems. In that moment, this book was born.

This is not a book about worms in chocolate. It is about learning to embrace food with pleasure. This is not a book about deprivation but about satisfaction. It is about journeying together to the "foul rag and bones shop of the heart" in order to uncover those forces that have kept you chained to bingeing, purging, chronic dieting, or starving. It is about discovering your own unique path to finally declaring peace with emotional eating.

Many years of my own life were taken up with the agony and the ecstasy of my relationship with food. Half of the time I spent sneaking food and bingeing. The other half of the time I was filled with repentance and would diligently watch my calories, weighing everything I ate on a postage scale so small it fit in my pocketbook.

Only when I began my own inner journey to understand and unravel my relationship with food did my recovery begin. In this journey I discovered that I was recruiting food to help me solve the emotional problems of living. I also came to recognize during the course of this journey that no chocolate chip cookie is smart enough to know how to truly comfort me. Today I eat with pleasure. I regard food as my friend and nourisher. But most of all, I have arrived at an inner peace with myself, my food and my body.

It was not always like this for me. As a child I loved food with an intense passion and always felt that I could never get enough good things to eat. When I was six years old, I wore a size 6X. The X meant I was too big for children's sizes that ended at just plain 6. It meant I was Xtra large, Xtra greedy, Xtra different from the other girls, and, therefore, should be Xtra ashamed of myself. I then went on to Chubby sizes and, since they down-scaled the numbers, I now wore a size 4. One time I bragged to one of my slender little classmates that I wore size 4. "Isn't that a Chubby size?" she asked innocently. I was mortified that it was so evident.

Now when I look at old pictures of myself, I see I really was not fat at all, although that was how I felt. I was plump, with dimples on my elbows, dark pigtails down my back, and I was cute.

I developed a needy relationship with food and began to sneak it. My mother would buy dessert and keep half of it, the next evening's portion, in our finished basement where it was nice and cool. My favorite were cakes with seven layers. I would go visit them and peek under the top of the bakery boxes. Pressing down the top of the cake, I would squish out the filling as layers from each of the seven strata would accumulate onto my finger, and I would lick them up. I could reduce a seven layer cake to practically a pancake in no time flat!

One evening, as my mother was preparing dinner, she burst into my room and demanded, "Who has been making inroads in the cake?" And since I was an only child and we had no dog and since my father was at work all day, I was obviously the culprit. To this day, the word "inroads" still strikes terror in my heart!

As a teenager, I cultivated other ways of sneaking food with the help of my house dress—the orange and the green one with snaps down the front and the big pockets. As my mother sat reading in the living room, I would saunter innocently into the kitchen "for a glass of water." I would turn on the faucet and carefully click open the refrigerator, seize my provisions, turn off the water tap, and proceed back to my room. Sometimes I added a cough to better camouflage the click of the refrigerator door.

Then there was the summer of my twelfth year when my parents and I went to Virginia for our summer vacation. Fearful I might not get enough to eat, I sneaked a jumbo package of *Good And Plenty* candy in the car with me. I popped them—like vitamins—trying not to jiggle the box too loudly from the back seat. Only years later did it dawn on me that I hated the taste of licorice, and I hated the pink and white candy coating. But that name, *Good And Plenty*! It captivated me. It meant that there would always be enough food for me and that I could always be in control.

My art of sneaking food developed further as I entered college and went to live with a family in Spain for my junior year abroad. One night when everyone was asleep, the craving to binge had me in its thrall, and I crept down the back stairway to where the cookies were kept in the Vera del Toro's pantry. In the darkness, I stuffed cookie after cookie into my mouth until I noticed with horror that at the far end of the kitchen was Yolanda, the thirteen-year-old daughter of the family with whom I lived. As we stared at each other, it dawned on me that I had walked in on *her* binge! We both stood looking at each other in humiliation. But, at the same time, this was a revelation to me. I had come thousands of miles across the ocean to discover something I had not known before—that I was not the only person in the world who binged and did strange, secretive things with food.

Returning home, I received my college degree and continued on to graduate school. One day a nice young man asked me to lunch, and that lunch became a turning point for me. I ordered a hamburger and, when it came, I had to bite my lip from crying because it was the smallest hamburger I had ever seen. My friend looked at me in confusion, "Are you all right? What's the matter?"

"This hamburger is so small," I blurted out despite myself and then blushed with embarrassment.

"Well, how about this," Aaron suggested kindly. "Why don't you eat this hamburger, and if you're still hungry when you've finished it, we'll order you another one."

I looked at him in astonishment. I realized he was suggesting something that I had never really thought of before—that when I am finished eating, I should take the time to check to see if I am still hungry, *and* if I am still hungry, I can always have more.

Strange as it may seem, before this incident I had never fully made the connection between physical hunger and eating. I ate at every chance I could regardless of whether I was physically hungry or not. This was because my passion for food and the tyrannical hold it had on me came from someplace deeper than just my stomach—it was a hunger deep from within my heart. And from that day on, I decided to open my heart and look at the experiences of my life which had led me to turn to food and which made me feel that trusting food was safer than trusting people. It was an inner journey of discovery that has changed my life. I no longer sneak cake filling, hoard *Good and Plenty* candy, or cry over small hamburgers.

Today, over twenty years since the beginning of my own journey, I am the director of The New York Center for Eating Disorders and have worked with hundreds of people to help them declare peace with their emotional eating. What I have learned is that each person's journey is as unique as a fingerprint. The complexity of eating disorders is such that no single cure works for all people. What works for one may not work for another.

For this reason, many people fail to resolve their eating problems because they keep trying to mold themselves to an approach that is not congruent with their inner self, their own true inner core. In *French Toast for Breakfast* we will work together to tailor an individualized approach that can work for you.

I should state at the outset that I strongly believe that social, cultural and political influences contribute to many eating problems, especially for women. A recent national women's magazine offers an unmistakable lesson in self-hatred: "Anorexics are taking over the world, and don't they look good! Thin has a better sex life, more boyfriends, a bigger house, a higher income than fat."[1]

Indeed, the constant pressure to be thin in today's society is extreme and provides a ripe context for the development of an eating disorder. But it is only when a person's own vulnerability is subjected to and absorbs these destructive cultural messages that a true eating problem develops. It is for this reason that I have chosen, in this book, to concentrate on the inner realm of the human heart where all true healing must begin.

French Toast for Breakfast is a book about *emotional eating*—being hungry from the heart, not from the stomach.

• Emotional eating is when you are lonely in the middle of the night and you look for comfort in the refrigerator.

• Emotional eating is when you are angry at somebody and you tear and chew into food when you are really wanting to bite that person's head off.

• Emotional eating is when you feel bored and empty and cannot figure out what to do for yourself, so you binge and make yourself vomit.

• Emotional eating is when you refuse to eat and starve yourself because you feel powerless and out-of-control over how your life is going.

• Emotional eating is using food to distract, detour, or deny your inner problems.

• Emotional eating is the domain of the compulsive eater, chronic dieter, bulimic and anorexic. Although each uses food in a different way—gorging, bingeing and purging, or starving—all are using food as a drug that can soothe, comfort, and keep them company or even punish and hurt them for their guilty feelings.

French Toast for Breakfast is also a book about *declaring peace with emotional eating and healing your eating problem*.

• Healing an eating problem means learning that food is not your enemy, that food was put on this earth to give you pleasure and to satisfy your hunger.

• True healing has to do with your *inner* state of mind. It means learning other nourishing ways of comforting and soothing yourself.

• Healing an eating problem means feeling at home in your body, treating it as a friendly ally rather than an object to be yelled at or criticized. This healing has little to do with thinness or fatness and can be achieved by people of all shapes and sizes.

• Healing an eating problem is about reclaiming the vitality of your inner self that has been hidden by your consuming relationship with food.

• Most of all, healing is about hope. It is about cultivating a deeply rich relationship with your inner self, your hunger for food and your hunger for life.

In Part I we will help you discover the root of your unique eating problem by exploring key underlying issues which include: The Fear of Fat, Shame and Intimacy, Sexuality, Anger, and the Fear of Success. Exercises called "Food for Thought" will follow each chapter to help you pinpoint the personal issues on which you will need to focus.

In Part II we will discuss how to create your own plan for peace by exploring various approaches for change. There are five tools for creating your own eating program: The Addictions Model, The No-Diet/No-Deprivation Approach, Habits, Psychotherapy, and Medication.

Part III includes a questionnaire to help you decide which approach or combination of approaches will work best for you. We will also discuss how to use a relapse as a launching pad for deeper recovery, and answer frequently-asked questions about healing an eating problem.

A word about the title: I have been struck by the number of my patients who have expressed to me a yearning for French toast for breakfast! They seldom satisfied this yearning because it seemed too much of a forbidden treat. My hope is that through this book, you will learn to make peace with all foods and begin to nurture yourself in other satisfying ways as well.

French Toast for Breakfast will help you sink your teeth into *life*—not into your obsession with food!

NOTE: Both men and women come to The New York Center for Eating Disorders. However, the majority are women. It is for this reason—and for simplicity in reading—that I use feminine pronouns throughout most of the book.

CHAPTER 1

The Fear of Fat
Decoding the Obsession

Whatever you can do, or think you can, begin it.
Boldness has genius, power and magic in it.
—Goethe

"Tell me what brings you here." I asked.

Brenda was a beautiful woman in her late thirties with long black hair and a slender body.

"Two months ago," she began, "I had a double mastectomy. And at that time my husband, Mark, left me for another woman. I realized he must have been seeing her a long time. My daughter, Sonia, the one who helped me through all this, is leaving next month for school in California. Now I have no one."

"And your family?" I asked.

"Both my parents are dead. They died in a car crash when I was twelve. Then I went to live with my grandmother. She died when I was 17. That's when I married Mark. Now I have no one."

She stared straight ahead, lost in reverie. The image of her parents' violent death, her mastectomies, and all her other losses was overwhelming.

"Brenda," I said, "you've been through so much. How would you like me to help you?"

She straightened up suddenly and said with determination, "I'm here because I'm fat and I need to lose weight!"

The language of pain comes in many dialects. Emotional eating problems and the fear of being fat is one such dialect in which we recruit our bodies to express what we cannot utter in words. Our eating problems become a vehicle to communicate matters of the heart that have no other channel. The language of food and fat is a symbolic one, a way to express our inner emotional battles over our feelings of emptiness and fullness, vulnerability and protection, urge and restraint, desire and despair.

When we cannot express the depth of pain we carry inside, we transform our emotional pain into physical pain. In the case of food problems, we move the focus from our heart to our stomach. We crystallize all our inner emotional pain into one concrete problem: "I am fat. I hate myself. I need to lose weight."

This is not to minimize the real upset that people feel when their eating is out of control. But what we are exploring here is the agony, self-hatred, and anxiety that rules the lives of many people when it comes to their bodies and their weight. This obsession with food and fat is often a shorthand way of expressing much deeper layers of yearning and pain.

Brenda, the woman whose story is recounted above, had been assaulted by so many massive losses in her life that she could not bear to face her grief, rage, and abandonment. Her wish to lose weight was a safe, clear way to express her pain—a language that so many people speak.

In this chapter we will try to decode this obsession with food and weight. We will try to translate the fear of being fat into its deeper meanings.

Why Are We Afraid of Fat?

Our culture is fat phobic. Fat people are degraded, discriminated against, pathologized and humiliated. When we take in this cultural message that fat lessens our worth and that thinness is a panacea, it becomes easy to subsume our many shortcomings under the rubric, "I am fat and ugly." If we do not identify what is truly bothering us, we fall prey to our own attacks on our fat — real or imagined. We camouflage our emotional problems by targeting our size.

Eating Styles and the Fear of Fat

Some clues as to the meaning behind the fear of being fat can be detected in the different eating styles of the anorexic, bulimic, or compulsive overeater.

The anorexic abhors her emotional neediness and so will starve herself as a way of proclaiming, "Look how strong I am. I have no needs. I don't need food. I don't need anyone. I have triumphed over my weaknesses and I am in control!"

The bulimic wavers back and forth between secret gorging rampages and violent purges of the food she has consumed. She purges to "repent" her neediness in the hopes of proclaiming, "I really can manage with very little. I'm able to give it back. I didn't mean to take it anyway." This oscillation between gorging and purging parallels her ambivalence about whether or not she deserves to take in nurturance and keep it.

For the overeater, the world never seems to offer enough sustenance. Her needs feel like they can never be satisfied. She does not trust in the abundance of food, just as she does not trust in the abundance of love and human kindness. She believes that it is safer to depend on food than on people. Food never leaves you, never rejects you, never laughs at you. And so, she attempts to take care of herself all by herself—just her and the food.

Developing the Fear of Fat

How does it come to pass that we divert our emotional problems into worries about our eating, fat and weight? How is it that a bodily function as natural as eating can take on such a complex myriad of meanings?

The field of psychosomatic medicine explores how we use different parts of our bodies to express our inner emotional states. We all know someone who suffers from a headache caused by inner tension, or a backache made worse by anger, or an ulcer triggered by stress. These psychosomatic problems are a physical way we try to cope with emotional conflicts which we cannot express directly. In this way, gorging, purging, starving, hating our bodies and fearing our fat can be viewed as outer manifestations of unexpressed inner feelings.

The Family Connection: Childhood Years

The connection between deep emotions and eating is a very understandable one. After all, our first introduction to the vital emotions of trust, dependency, security, generosity, love and the acceptability of our needs starts at birth in the feeding experience with our parents. Even the capacity to love has its origins in the satisfaction of being well nourished. Anna Freud coined the term "stomach love" to describe the baby's early attachment to the parents who feed it.

If our parents are attuned to our feeding needs when we are babies and children, if they let us set the pace and rhythm, if they let us initiate and control the feeding relationship, then we learn that our needs are important and we feel a security with the world. And if our parents continue to read our hunger cues correctly, we ourselves learn how to identify and respond correctly to our hunger cues as we grow.

Of course, not every parent is exquisitely attuned at every moment in every feeding situation. Parents catch colds, feel irritable, have car trouble. In fact, our parents only need to be "good enough" to set us on the road to growth. A mother or father who is too indulgent will over gratify us, and we will never learn to tolerate frustration. But if our parents are "good enough," if our connection to them is bountiful enough, we are left with a sense of contentment in our relationship to them, to our food and to our bodies.

On the other hand, when a parent uses food repeatedly as a pacifier to keep us quiet, as a reward for good behavior, or as a punishment by withholding food when we are "bad," then food becomes a tool to control us. We then begin to connect eating with reward and punishment. We lose the sense that eating is really about hunger. And just as our parents may incorrectly decode our hunger signals, we start decoding them incorrectly as well—fatigue means I should eat, anxiety means I should binge and throw up, anger means I should starve.

This confusion of signals is captured with frightening accuracy by author Carol Hill, as she describes the destructive interaction between a mother and son over food. In this vignette, the mother has come to pick up her son, Francis, from school.

> "You must be hungry," she said. "I brought you a piece of home-made cake," and with one hand steering she shoved a chocolate layer cake on a green paper plate, covered with wax paper, across the seat to Francis.
>
> "I, I coulda waited until we got home," Francis said, uncomfortable at being baited.
>
> "Well, yes," the high pitch came back. "I know you could have, I was just trying to be *nice*." The high note pierced his ear. "You don't have to eat it dear, but be sure to wipe your hands. I don't want chocolate all over the seats."
>
> And Francis felt again the old vortex rising, "Obey, don't obey, do, don't eat, not, spill not, mess not, wipe not, be not," and he sucked an extra long time on a chocolate crumb-encased finger.[1]

The Family Connection: Teenage Years

Most people who come to see me for eating disorder therapy began to be afraid of fat during their teenage years. At this time, the developmental tasks of adolescence often get detoured into an increasing obsession with food and body size.

If all has gone "good enough" between parent and child with feeding and emotional attunement, the teenager will enter adolescence—the time of greatest self-image and body change—with relative smoothness. A father will stay connected to his daughter when confronted with her developing body and budding sexuality, not leaving the girl to feel abandoned. A mother will also stay connected, not becoming competitive or overly critical of this emerging young woman. Then the girl will experience pleasure that her body is beginning to resemble her mother's.

But, sadly, this is not always the case and the numerous conflicts a girl may have had with her parents and with becoming female get displaced onto her own body. The ever-shifting battle with her mother—to stay connected and become like her on one hand and to separate and become independent of her on the other hand—often leaves the girl confused. Her relationship with her father is also changing dramatically, leaving behind the security of being Daddy's little girl. The energy needed to negotiate this important passage from childhood to womanhood can easily get derailed into obsessing about her body.

To understand the meanings behind emotional eating problems, we need to come to terms with our femaleness and with the identification with our mothers' bodies which "we have raged against...yearned for...been tormented by its absence, stood in mortal need of its closeness, thought of it as fate, felt it as destiny, and knew it to be world." [2]

As a teenager, Ellen struggled with many of these issues. Her mother was crippled with arthritis when she was born, and as a result, was unable to hold or feed the baby for long periods of time. Mrs. Lawson would prop Ellen up on a pillow by herself with the bottle in her mouth. As she grew older, she was also left alone in the high chair for long periods of time to feed herself. Because Mrs. Lawson was increasingly bedridden and overwhelmed by her husband's heavy drinking, Ellen was forced to come home right after school each day to act as her mother's nurse and confidante.

During Ellen's childhood, Mrs. Lawson required many hospitalizations, and Ellen comforted herself through the night by overeating. By the time she was a teenager, she weighed over two hundred pounds. Her closest moments with her mother were when the two of them joined forces and went on a diet together. It was during these dieting episodes that Ellen felt the most connected to and cared for by her mother.

By the time Ellen reached adolescence, she was caught in a struggle of enormous magnitude. She wanted a life of her own with friends her own age, but she felt tremendous guilt leaving her mother for even a single afternoon. The tension of choosing whether to go out with friends or meet her obligations to her mother caused Ellen to gorge on food and then make herself throw up. By age twenty, she was deeply entrenched in a pattern of bulimia.

She came to therapy at age twenty-two, not to talk about her pain with her family nor the dangers of being bulimic, but because she was in a rage at not being able to lose weight. "If only I weren't so fat, the boys would ask me out."

Ellen's fear of being fat was her shorthand way of expressing how torn apart she felt about whether she was entitled to be separate from her mother. Following a particularly fierce episode of bingeing and purging, she related a dream which connected her bulimia to this confusion and guilt she felt towards her mother. "I was standing over the toilet bowl and I was puking. I saw my mother's head in the bowl. I couldn't move. I just stood there paralyzed. I didn't know what to do, whether to flush the toilet with her in it or fish her out."

What we uncovered in this violent dream were Ellen's murderous feelings towards her mother which had been submerged in her eating problem. Ellen's binge was an attempt to soothe anxiety, to join and connect with her mother, even to "eat" her mother to protect her from Ellen's rage. (As strange as that may sound, there is a cannibalistic aspect to eating disorders. After all, eating is the earliest way we have to take in our mothers and keep them inside of ourselves. It has been pointed out that mother is "one who gives her own body to be eaten. She first nourished the child in her womb and then gives it her milk."[3])

Her binge had another meaning, as well. Ellen was angrily and cruelly chewing and tearing her mother to pieces for making Ellen her sole life support. In purging, Ellen was trying to undo this rage, purify herself of this anger, and restore her mother unharmed from the aggression. Throwing up was also her way to punish herself for feeling like such a murderous daughter in the first place.

As we slowly unraveled these meanings, Ellen's bulimia and fear of fat began to ebb. Her therapy provided her an opportunity—for the first time in her life—to verbalize her pain and anger rather than swallow it, and to purge the guilt she had felt for so many years.

Decoding the Meaning

Our fear of fat is a signal that there is a unique message yearning to emerge from our inner self, and for this reason, we can use our obsession with food by "milking" it for the meanings it offers us for self-discovery. We need to uncover that inner message, decode and understand it, and use it to heal ourselves. Rather than grouping all our needs under the generic, "I am fat and need to lose weight," we must tease out the varieties, nuances, and subtleties of what our deep emotions really are. Do I want to be taken care of? Do I want to be held? Do I need to rest? We can even look at how our fat phobia, at times, has actually "helped us" negotiate our fears and anxieties.

As we try to decode the specific meanings behind a person's fear of fat, we usually find that at the heart of the matter is some form of struggle about conflicting feelings having to do with neediness, with family relationships, and with rage and guilt.

Neediness

People with eating problems often feel their emotional needs are repulsive and see their bodies as the external symbol for these shameful inner needs. "If I can control my body," they think, "then I can control my emotional neediness." Actually, many have no idea what their needs really are because everything has become so detoured through food. Others mistakenly consider their need for nurturing as selfish.

One patient of mine, Amy, had learned in her family that it was easier to overeat than to risk the humiliation of asking anyone for anything. Her family had always made her feel like a "baby" and a "whiner" when she asked for their help or support.

One day she came to her therapy session with a bloody finger. She had just cut herself on her car door and hated to bother me by taking the band-aid I offered. The following week she left a large box of brand new band-aids in my bathroom. In our next session, I asked why she felt obligated to replace the one band-aid I had given her with a full box. Amy admitted she always feared her needs were a drain on the people she cared about, so she always tried to make it up to them—as she was now doing with me. Later, she would make it up to herself by gorging on food.

Family Separation

Anxiety and guilt about separating from one's parents or doing better than they have done is another issue which frequently underlies a person's emotional eating.

Judith came to therapy saying she felt trapped by her large body. Although she was happily married, financially well-off, and had two healthy children, she claimed her weight was the major obstacle preventing her from taking pleasure in her life. In exploring the reasons for this, Judith realized, "I always felt inadequate because I could never make my mother happy. I thought that if I could first heal her pain, then I would feel entitled to go after my own dreams. But I always felt that my happiness was like salt in my mother's wounds, and she's already suffered enough."

Judith explained, "My mother was born in Germany and when she was sixteen, the Nazis rounded up the Jews in her village and herded them into concentration camps. Once there, the Nazis divided the Jews into two lines, one to be killed and one to be put to work. My mother was ill, so she was put on the line to die. But when the Nazi guard wasn't looking, she ran to the other line. Then the most horrible thing happened. The guard realized the lines were uneven, so he plucked a girl from the survivor group and placed her on the line to be gassed. And so my mother survived at the expense of another girl's life. For the rest of her life she felt responsible for killing that girl. She tortured herself endlessly, never going on vacation, never buying nice clothes for herself. By just surviving, she felt guilty."

The guilt Mrs. Stern felt at "killing" someone to save herself was visited on her daughter each time Judith would strive to be happy. No! She couldn't take ballet lessons—no one in concentration camp ever had ballet lessons. No! She couldn't have a sweet sixteen party—no one in concentration camp ever had a sweet sixteen party. But Judith, who was born in the United States and was full of life, wanted all these things and more.

Then sometime after her sixteenth birthday—the same age her mother had "sent" someone to her death—Judith developed a compulsive overeating problem. She just got fatter and fatter. Every time she would enjoy herself, whether it was ice skating with her girlfriends or having a good time at a party, she would gorge and gorge to make herself desperate and miserable. This pattern continued throughout her life. If she planned a vacation with her husband, she would negate the pleasure of this anticipated trip by bingeing on food. If she was promoted on her job, she would gain ten pounds to undo the pleasure of this success. Every step Judith took to be happy felt like a betrayal of the bond of pain she shared with her mother, who was also unhappy about her own large size. So, Judith abused food and her body to insure that happiness would never be hers.

"I'm betraying my mother if I give myself things and make myself happy. I'm not allowed to have it all. When I do enjoy myself, I begin to overeat, get fat, and make myself miserable to 'even the score.' I should know my place."

"And what place is that?" I asked. Judith fell silent.

The night after my question, she had this dream: "I was waiting on line at the supermarket check-out counter and saw I could get out faster if I pushed ahead of an older woman on the next line. I ran in front of her and knocked her down. She was hurt and started crying. I paid for my groceries—all cakes and cookies—and ran to the car to devour them."

The dream revealed that as Judith desired to push ahead in life, she also felt she was abandoning her mother and sending her mother to the line of suffering and pain. Judith saw herself as a greedy murderer, as if her success had the power to rob her mother of a companion in suffering. Judith was reliving the survivor guilt her mother felt towards the girl in the concentration camp. Only through gorging and hating her fat could she "keep herself in line." Judith's eating problem became a prison that was her punishment for wishing to break free.

"Somewhere deep in the fiber of my being, I believe I have to honor my mother's pain. She always hated herself for being fat. If I share this with her, at least maybe she won't be so alone in that way," Judith concluded.

Such is the intimate bond with our parents that it can lead us to sacrifice ourselves in order to relieve their pain. An eating disorder can be a way of stating to them and to ourselves, "I will never leave you. I hope my suffering and sacrifice will redeem you and make you happy. Then maybe later it will be my turn for happiness."

The sad truth, of course, is that we cannot undo the past suffering of our parents. In time, through therapy, Judith began to see this. She was able to bring her conflicted feelings out into the clear light of day where she could then understand and begin to overcome them. She realized that beneath her fixation with her weight lay the much larger issue of survivor guilt—the belief that achieving success meant a betrayal of her mother. Slowly, as her anxiety diminished, she could then focus on her appetite for life, pleasure, and success.

Rage and Guilt

Suppressed rage which has no direct avenue of expression is another frequent cause of an obsession with food and weight.

Karen was filled with self-disgust at what she felt was her "fat and ugly body" and would accuse herself unmercifully of being a bad person when she binged. Like so many people who suffer from emotional eating, Karen was actually transforming an intensely difficult personal experience in her life into the familiar pain about body size. Familiar pain is more endurable than anguish over which we have no control.

Karen was a twin and was always more lively and outgoing than her sister, Laurie. Growing up twins, they had their own special language and often dressed alike. But as the two of them grew older, Karen increasingly found her twinship to be a burden. At times Laurie seemed like a lost soul who described her life as "being in a boat in the middle of a lake without any oars." And her dependency on Karen—such as her wish to tag along with Karen's friends—was such a responsibility that, at times, Karen secretly wished she were not a twin so she could just be her own person. This wish made her feel guilty for being so selfish.

When Laurie and Karen were twenty-two years old, Laurie killed herself. In her suicide note she told of years of bitter unhappiness and severe doubts about herself. Karen was devastated. She blamed herself because she should have known how desperate her twin had been. What tormented her even more, though, was the conviction that it was her own desire to be more separate that had killed Laurie.

In the first part of Karen's therapy, we came to understand that her incessant self-hatred about her fat was really a cover-up for her guilt over her sister's death.

In the second part of her therapy, we realized that Karen's yelling at herself for being "fat and ugly" was her way of turning the rage she felt towards Laurie against herself. Karen condemned her eating and fat with words like, "selfish, only thinking about myself, just interested in my own needs." In truth, this was how she felt about Laurie's selfish disregard for the shattered lives she had left behind.

Karen came to understand and accept her rage and slowly began to forgive herself for feeling this way. As she forgave herself, she felt less of a need for emotional eating. By going through the process of uncovering the layers beneath the surface of her relationship with food, she eventually was able to declare peace with her eating problems.

Decoding as a First Step Towards Resolution

Decoding our fear of fat is the first step towards resolving our emotional eating, because once we identify what we need and feel, we can then determine how we are going to express those needs directly without recruiting our bodies to do it for us. The more we can cultivate a rich vocabulary to express our inner emotional selves and the more we can cultivate a deep responsiveness to our inner needs, the less likely we will speak the language of fat and pain.

Decoding our fear of fat will help us release the energy and power to unfold our most genuine selves—needy and strong, vulnerable and independent, humorous and serious, and all the colors in between!

Food for Thought Exercises

These exercises will help you identify how the fear of fat may be an obstacle in healing your eating problem. Use your answers as a springboard to deepen your own self-knowledge.

1. Are you obsessed by a fear of fat? How long have you felt this way?

2. Are there any patterns you can detect? Did these obsessions arise in response to separation, guilt, anger, sexuality?

3. What is your fat phobia distracting you from in your current life?

4. If your fat (real or imagined) had a voice, to whom would it speak and what would it say?

5. What in your history has made it hard for you to claim your needs directly?

CHAPTER 2

Shame and Intimacy

*You're fat and ugly and
your mother dresses you funny.*
—Bumper sticker
Brooklyn, New York

Each summer of the years I was in grade school, I tried to lose weight in anticipation of the day I would have to go shopping for back-to-school clothes. I was nine when my aunt took me on one of these shopping trips, and none of the clothes fit. At one point we took a break to have lunch, and because I was afraid of getting hungry later in the afternoon, I asked her to wrap up my leftover muffin and take it with us. We returned to another unsuccessful round of shopping when my aunt, in a burst of frustration, turned to the saleswoman, opened her pocketbook and revealed my muffin. "Look how much she eats!" she said. "I even have to carry food around for her!" Tears of shame welled up inside of me and then froze. I thought I was a bad, unlovable child—unlike other children who would never dream of asking anyone to carry a muffin in their pocketbook.

From my years of working with individuals, families, and groups, I have discovered that at the root of many eating problems lies an underlying emotion we seldom recognize. It is often more basic and more powerful than the emotions usually associated with eating disorders such as anger, fear, or loneliness. It is often the key dynamic that propels people to binge, to vomit, or to starve. It is shame.

Anyone who is an emotional eater is no stranger to shame—shame about how insatiable we can feel at our core, shame about what lengths we have gone to get food, and shame for the secret gorging rampages that override reason. Our most intense fear is that what we do in secret with food will be found out, and we will be exposed to ridicule because then everyone will know how greedy we really are.

This deep inner sense of shame can drive us to the temporary comfort of a relationship with food. In the case of emotional eating, though, the painful paradox is that overeating, starving or purging, which we originally turned to for relief of our shameful feelings, turn on us in time and become a source of shame in their own right. The very method we used to help ourselves with pain begins to generate its own pain and shame.

People are often confused about the difference between shame and guilt. Actually, they are similar in that they both contribute to our feeling bad about ourselves, but they differ in emphasis. We feel guilty for something we *do* or for harboring some "bad" thought. A guilty person thinks, 'I shouldn't have done that," or "I shouldn't think that way." Shame, on the other hand, is about feeling deficient or defective in the core of our being—our inner self. The shameful person feels, "I am ashamed of my *self*. I shouldn't *be* that way."

The Origins of Shame

Shame can come to live inside us for many reasons, but most often because of the influences of our family, our peer group, and our culture. Children, eager for approval, are particularly vulnerable to critical remarks from their parents or siblings. Teenagers, who also have an enormous need for acceptance among their peers, know that any deviation—especially as it relates to appearance—can result in their being ridiculed or ostracized. Finally, in today's culture, fashion models and movie stars continue to be held up as the "standard," and women are judged by their appearance. This plays an on-going role in generating shame.

Family Shame

Ideally, each of us has parents who love us unconditionally. Certainly they do not have to gratify us all the time, but we should feel that we can depend on them to respect, acknowledge, and respond to our needs as they arise. If we grow up in a family where we are made to feel ashamed of these needs and wants, our real self goes into hiding.

> "When one feels empty inside, hungry to feel a part of someone, desperate to be held close, craving to be wanted and admired, respected and loved—but these have become taboo through shame—one turns instead to food. But food can never truly satisfy the inner need. Longing turns to shame. And so one eats more to anesthetize the longing."[1]

An occasional experience of being shamed will not, of course, be responsible for a child internalizing shameful feelings. We are speaking here of a *pattern* of response—

the habitual experience of being humiliated in our families of origin. If we cannot show our neediness because of our fear of ridicule, or show our hurt and pain because we will be laughed at, or if our hunger for emotional connection is derided, we may turn instead toward food.

Rebecca, a client of mine, described how food became her source of comfort when her feelings were denied. "When I was ten, I had to be in a special children's hospital for several months recovering from an operation. My parents could only visit me on weekends, and I would cry every Sunday night when they had to leave. I begged them to take me home, and they yelled at me for not appreciating everything they were doing to make me better. I felt guilty and ashamed for not being more thankful. I was so lonely when they left, and I remember feeling that the shopping bag of food they brought was my only link to them. I even went to sleep one night with a loaf of Italian bread in the hospital bed with me. At least for the moment the food took away my feelings that I was a bad, ungrateful child."

Parents are more likely to make their children feel ashamed of having needs if they themselves are facing stressful life situations, such as a family member who is physically or emotionally ill, financial worries, or trouble in their marriage. At these times, they will find their child's needs and emotions to be an extra, unwanted demand. The burdened parent, in turn, often responds to their child with ridicule, contempt, dismissal, or anger. These shaming responses can set in motion the child's attempt to cover up her real feelings by portraying a make-believe self to the outside world and hiding behind food for comfort.

Vivian described in one therapy session how her parents made her feel ashamed for being afraid. "Cookies became my whole life when I was seven. I even remember the day. My parents were both drinking at the time. When I got home from school there were moving men packing us up! My parents had never told me we were going to move. I started crying but Dad said, 'Stop that! You shouldn't feel upset. We're moving somewhere you'll like even better.' His tone was so sharp that I remember feeling something must be wrong with me for being upset. Dad's reaction made me ashamed that I had doubted him. That day I ate a whole box of shortbread cookies which became my security blanket. Even now, 25 years later, when someone chides me with 'you shouldn't feel that way,' I run to the cookies to hide myself because I assume they must be right. The really sad part is not only am I ashamed for what I'm feeling but also for how much I overate!"

Ashamed for crying

In my work with eating disorder patients, I have repeatedly seen how inner prohibitions against crying can be very strong. Parents, hoping to prevent their child from suffering or if they themselves are uncomfortable with crying, will scold or shame a child away from tears. For many bulimics, vomiting is a substitute for crying. In situations where other people cry, bulimics throw up. The vomiting makes them feel less vulnerable because they can control their purges, and they do not always have that power over unbidden tears.

Parents shame their children by saying:
"Don't cry—here's a lollipop."
"Big girls don't cry."

"If you don't stop, I'll really give you something to cry about."

"Stop it! You know how your crying upsets your mother."

"You're such a crybaby. When are you going to grow up?"

"You're making a mountain out of a molehill."

"Don't be a sissy —boys don't cry."

"You should be ashamed of yourself for carrying on like this."

"When I was your age, I really had something to cry about."

"You're just oversensitive."

"You can cry to your heart's content but it won't get you anywhere."

"Your brother never went on and on like you do."

"Go to your room and don't come out until you're done crying."

"Your crying will be the death of me."

"Why in the world are you crying? There's nothing to cry about."

What we find is that stifling tears leads to furtive eating, secret purging, or starving out the pain.

Ashamed for being selfish

Children who are made to feel that their wishes are selfish often find relief in bingeing, purging or starving.

Emily: "I feel like such a bad and selfish person. A friend of mine just had a mastectomy, and she calls me late in the evening because she's depressed. By that hour I'm exhausted, and when we are done talking, there is no time left over for me. I find myself bingeing and then going to sleep. How can I tell her not to call when she is going through such a rough time? If I were ever in her situation, I'd want to know I could count on my friends."

"In discussing this with my support group, I realized that because of my fear of being selfish, I have been giving too much of myself. The food 'helps' me keep my mouth shut in situations where I should be speaking up. This is such a direct parallel with my upbringing. My grandmother lived with us the last three years before she died, and the whole household stopped to cater to her. Whenever I wanted to have friends over or play music, my father would say, 'You should be ashamed of yourself. You're so selfish. Don't you realize Grandma's sick? Someday that might be you.' For me to say 'no' means being selfish, but I'm learning that unless I assert my limitations, stuffing down food becomes my 'solution.'"

Ashamed for being needy

Children who are made to feel ashamed of their natural human needs will often try to satisfy these needs through a relationship with food.

Charlotte: "In my family there was always competition for who was the thinnest and who had the strongest personality. Even to rest or relax is considered a weakness in my family. To this day, my mother, who is retired, feels obliged to comment, 'I was so busy today—I didn't even have time to sit down once!'"

"My whole life has felt like a performance—pushing myself to be the best in everything. When I'm into starving myself or using laxatives, I feel triumphant, as if I have no needs and I'm totally in control. But everything fell apart when my husband left me. Even though I was devastated, my parents kept telling me, 'You're a Franklin. We Franklins can make it on our own. We don't need anybody.' I was ashamed that for the first time I couldn't get out of bed, I couldn't stop crying, and I couldn't stop eating. It was like a dam had burst, and all my years of pretending to be strong started to crumble. I'm also ashamed that I had to go for therapy. My parents would practically disown me if they knew, but I just don't have the energy left to act as if I don't need anything or anybody."

Ashamed for how you look

Children who feel used as an ornament by their parents come to believe that their real selves are not good enough to make their parents proud. This can set up a child's need to find comfort through food.

Pamela: "My mother always wanted a curly, blonde-haired daughter. One summer, when I was 13, she dyed my hair blonde and gave me a permanent. When I went to junior high school in the fall, she told me not to tell anyone it wasn't my real color or style. She also taught me how to glue on false eyelashes and told me to keep that a secret, too. I went along with her. I guess I believed that my hair was not that great, but I also remember feeling ashamed that I wasn't pretty enough for her to love me just the way I was. I gained a lot of weight when I was in junior high, which only added to my feeling of never being good enough."

Ashamed for feeling anger or hate

If children are given the message that anger is unacceptable, they can discharge this emotion through bingeing, purging, or starving rather than expressing it directly.

Gail: "I was born with a harelip and had to go to doctors all the time. I hated it. I would cry and scream until my father retaliated with, 'You should be grateful. We don't even have the money to be doing what we're doing for you!' But I hated those doctor visits so much, and I hated my parents for forcing me to go."

"It was only years later that I realized the impact his words had on me. I was in a terrible marriage and had gained 80 pounds. After coming to therapy for awhile, I realized that the reason I got involved with Ben, even though I knew he was unfaithful, was that I was so grateful that anyone would want me with this deformed lip. My eating was stuffing down the guilt I felt for hating him. I also didn't feel I had any *right* to be angry. Only now am I beginning to accept how hurt and scared I was as a child and how ashamed I felt about the harelip. In my therapy group, I'm learning to feel more *entitled* to my anger. The more justified I feel about my anger, the less I need the food to help me squelch myself."

Ashamed for trying to comfort oneself

The eminent British child analyst, D.W. Winnicott, discusses how "security blankets" (a doll, a stuffed toy, special pajamas) are objects that help children make the transition between running to their parents for comfort and being able to soothe themselves. This capacity to comfort ourselves in moments of distress or pain that we learn in childhood becomes a rich, inner resource in adult life when we are sad or lonely or hurting.

Where there is a breach in the parents' ability to respond with empathy, there will also be a breach in the child's ability to soothe himself. Rather than appreciating the "security blanket" stage as a healthy part of development, parents may feel annoyed by the "babyishness" of it and discourage or humiliate the child with phrases like, "When are you going to grow up?" "Big boys don't play with dolls." "Take your thumb out of your mouth." Parents may simply throw out the blanket or toy, much to the child's grief. The child is then cheated of the pleasure and assurance of knowing how to soothe his own needs, and food becomes his pacifier instead.

Ashamed into believing image is more important than one's inner self

When children do not feel loved unconditionally, they often retreat into a relationship with food.

David: "It seemed like making a good impression was my mother's driving motivation, and I never truly felt that I could get her approval. My father's drinking made her especially worried about what the neighbors would think."

"I was always good in sports and had won many trophies. My mother had shelves built in my bedroom to show them off to other people, but she never really told me that *she* was proud of me. I thought she took all the glory for herself when the neighbors came over, and at the same time, I was ashamed for always craving her approval. I was left feeling hollow inside—very unappreciated—and the jelly donuts were my way of making it up to myself."

Ashamed for being sexual

Parents are often threatened by children's sexual play and exploration. Children who are made to feel ashamed of their bodies in their early years grow up uncomfortable with their sexuality as adults. Emotional eating can be a way to bypass these sexual feelings.

Marie: "When I was ten, I was squatting on the floor with a mirror under me to get a better look at my vagina. My mother caught me and started to laugh. She told my father, and they kidded me for a long time after that. I felt so ashamed and betrayed."

June: "My older sister found me and my cousin Jim playing doctor. We were undressed, and she ran to tell my aunt who slapped me. She told me that was 'dirty play' and 'nice girls didn't do that.' She never scolded my cousin though. I learned the message that girls shouldn't have feelings 'down there.' No wonder I'm 60 pounds overweight!"

In many troubled families, children are often the victims of sexual abuse—the ultimate betrayal of trust that a child can experience. The scars of sexual abuse are further complicated by feelings of guilt for complying with the abuser—not recognizing that as a child, there are often no alternatives. Shame can be particularly strong if one is aware of having enjoyed the contact. Bingeing, purging, or starving then becomes a way of suppressing "shameful" sexual energy as well as hiding from sexual intimacy.

Ashamed for being a child and forced into being a parent

Children are needy by nature, and parents who ridicule and shame their vulnerability send the message that it is not all right to be a dependent child. Children may even find themselves receiving more parental love and approval for being their parents' caretaker. "She's five going on 25. She's mother's little helper." Addictions and compulsive behavior are often an attempt, albeit unsuccessful, to nurture one's self on one hand, and to deny one's need for nurturance on the other.

Roberta: "I was the second oldest girl of eight kids. My father was not working steadily, and I was frightened by how worried and depressed my mother was. I kept thinking that if only I could help her more she would be happier—that it was up to me. I cooked, I cleaned, I took my brothers and sisters to school. I would do anything I could to take care of my mother. My role in the family was to be needed, and my whole sense of worth was based on that."

"This really hit home when I was 18. I was holding down two jobs and one day walked by a neighborhood deli with a big sign in the window: 'Needed: part-time cashier.' I went right in. The word 'needed' magnetized me because if someone had a need, I automatically thought I should take care of it! I see now how my drinking and bulimia have been my attempt to refuel myself, rather than realizing that *I* need someone to take care of *me* sometimes, too."

Ashamed for not being perfect enough

For parents who want their children to be perfect, nothing is ever good enough. Many of my patients have described bringing home report cards from school with grades of 90%, only to be ridiculed, "What happened to the other ten points?" Emotional eaters use food to assuage their disappointment, fear, and rage at not meeting their parents' standards.

Lois: "My family had strong religious values. I was always being criticized for not having enough humility and for having too much pride. They always reminded me that 'pride comes before the fall' whenever I'd express some excitement about being chosen class president or making the school swim team. In my home and in my particular Church we were taught to devote our lives to "J.O.Y."—Jesus first, Others second, and Yourself third. Through my therapy, I came to realize that my anorexia was about trying to disown all my needs—hunger included—to make myself a more perfect little girl in the eyes of my family. Now my goal is "Y.O.J." in which "Yourself" goes first! Unless I put myself first and focus on my own recovery, I won't be any good for Others or for Jesus! I will remain that skinny girl who keeps trying to starve herself to be more and more perfect."

Ashamed for wanting to be separate and different from one's family

Parents who need their child to be dependent on them in order to feel important will make that child feel guilty and ashamed for her wish to grow up and be separate. The parent communicates, "What would I do without you?" "How could you leave me after all I've done for you?" "You are my whole life." "I've always sacrificed myself for you." The child will use emotional eating as a way of staying connected to the parent out of guilt (compulsive overeating), wishing to eject the parent out of her system (bulimia), or starving the parent's messages out of her body (anorexia).

I was witness to a vivid and painful illustration of this connection between emotional eating and a child's conflict over separating. While riding a bus I noticed a mother and her obese daughter of about 13 sitting across from me, and I commented to myself that the girl looked like a baby elephant. No sooner did I think that when the mother took out a bag of peanuts, began shelling them for her daughter, and popping them into the girl's waiting mouth. The girl sat there, miserable yet passive. Mama's feeding had become a controlling and powerful bond which tied her daughter to her. The girl's need to separate from her mother was literally being trunk-ated!

Peer Shame

Families are not the only medium for generating shame. If the seeds of shame have been planted in the child's early years, they often emerge in full bloom during adolescence when the pressure for peer group approval becomes very important. Many emotional eaters have felt deeply shamed by their peers if they look or act different in any way. Being chosen last for team sports or being forced to be weighed in front of one's classmates are painful experiences. Being the "90 pound weakling" fills a teenage boy with shame as does being the young teenage girl who has not begun to develop like her friends. Shame begets shame, and emotional eating begets further emotional eating.

Cultural Shame

Although the seeds of shame can be planted within our families of origin, families are often acting upon the prevailing cultural attitudes of the day. Parents—like all of us—are vulnerable to these hurtful cultural messages about size, image, needs and self-worth, and they can communicate these messages to their children.

It has been said that "a culture is a family's family," and certainly in our westernized culture, women have been shamed for being anything other than an ideal— thin, quiet, and non-assertive. In the same way that families can negate children's needs, our culture tends to deny that women have needs, feelings, or appetites.

A New York radio announcer embodies this cultural message when he greets his radio audience each day with, "Good morning, listeners, and especially you, size nine." "Size nine" is nonchalantly reduced from being a woman with thoughts, feelings, and desires to a mere object. She is also set apart from all those other women who are (shamefully) *not* "size nine."

Shame as a Vicious Cycle

As adults, feeling ashamed can continue to fuel our emotional eating, and we develop a "shame cycle" that keeps us locked into a fixed pattern.

Victor, a patient of mine who struggled with compulsive eating, described the efforts he made to suppress his anger toward his elderly father. "Dad is always getting on my nerves by directing me and criticizing me for how I should run my business. But he's really such a nice guy. He wouldn't hurt a fly." Often Victor's anger and frustration broke through and he would start screaming at his father. He would then feel ashamed for having "lost it," eat to try to calm down, and then eat again to help him suppress his anger once more. His cycle looked like this:

ANGRY OUTBURST

SUPPRESSED ANGER   SHAME FOR ANGER

OVEREATING TO   OVEREATING TO
RELIEVE SHAME   CONSOLE HIMSELF

SHAME FOR EATING

Claire had another version of the shame cycle. As the oldest of seven children, she learned to swallow and deny any of her needs because they were too overwhelming for her parents to deal with. Any feeling or need that she experienced led her immediately to feel ashamed. Claire identified these patterns:

LONGING FOR ATTENTION ➡ SHAME ➡ FOOD ➡PURGING
ANGER ➡ SHAME ➡ FOOD ➡ PURGING
JEALOUSY ➡ SHAME ➡ FOOD ➡ PURGING
SEXUAL FEELINGS ➡ SHAME ➡ FOOD ➡ PURGING

The Toll of Shame

The most devastating effect of chronic shaming is that it creates within us a fear of intimacy. We come to believe that food is safer than relationships. As one patient described, "If people knew the real me—how greedy I am inside—they would leave me because I'm so unlovable." Other emotional eaters may project their neediness onto others and worry, "If I get close to you, maybe *your* neediness will eat me up alive and I'd have to run away from you!" We distort in various ways:

"I must be unlovable," becomes "I don't need love."

"I don't need love," becomes "I don't want love."

"I don't want love," becomes "I will reject love when it comes because there is no such thing; I cannot trust it, it's not safe."

"I don't need love, I don't want love," ultimately becomes "I won't take love, I can't take it!" [2]

Then our obsessive relationship with food becomes the path of least resistance.

Recovering from Shame

The first step in recovering from an eating problem caused by shame is to acknowledge that shameful feelings exist within us. This will help us begin to identify those painful family experiences that, up to now, have gone nameless even though they lived in the pit of our stomachs. By exposing these experiences to the clear light of our awareness, we begin to see how they caused us to mistrust and fear relationships with people and caused us to turn instead to a relationship with food.

After becoming aware of our shameful feelings, we must begin to undo our inner prohibitions as well as our family's prohibitions against expressing our feelings. "It is not the traumas we suffer in childhood that make us emotionally ill, but the inability to express the trauma." [3] When we can reveal our genuine feelings both to ourselves and to others, the process of healing is set in motion.

The Healing Power of Relationships

Coming out of hiding involves reaching out to others. We cannot heal our shame alone. Just as hurtful relationships were the cause of our turning to food in the first place, so will supportive and loving relationships be the medium of our healing.

We must connect with other people who can validate our pain, our rejections, our hurt, and accept us for who we are. In this way, through a support group or through therapy, we create a "second chance" family. When we realize that this new family accepts the parts of ourselves we have "discarded" because of shame, we learn to accept ourselves as well.

Building trust in new relationships is a slow process. We are asking ourselves to take the leap to reveal and expose our inner shameful feelings, while all our lifelong efforts have been to hide and cover up. As Charles Whitfield so poignantly describes in *Healing the Child Within*, "Recovery is about telling the story of our suffering to safe and supportive others. What we expose and share is our Child Within, our True Self with all its weaknesses and all of its strengths. We need others to help us heal ourselves. They validate our predicaments and our pain and they accept us as we are. And when we hear others tell their stories and share their shame, we help them to heal."[4]

When she was 15, Vickie had been deeply shamed by her father for her budding sexual interest in boys. He had caught her kissing a boy on their porch and let her know in no uncertain terms that she was a whore. He repeated this message so unrelentingly that this shame came to live inside Vickie. She became fatter and fatter, and the rest of her teenage years were spent in retreat from those early, dangerous sexual feelings.

When Vickie began therapy with me and had some success gaining control of her binge eating, she became worried that I was secretly judging and criticizing her. We discovered that when her weight subsided as *the issue* in her life, feelings of wanting a relationship with a man emerged. She began to feel that if she became sexual, I too would see her as a whore and would roundly disapprove of her interest in the opposite sex.

The shame she had internalized from her father's disapproval was now coming alive again in our relationship as she unconsciously externalized it onto me. This gave her an opportunity to relive with me, in the role of her disapproving father, the memories and pain stored within her all these years—the pain that had been hidden by her eating and her weight. The relationship with me, however, did not repeat the pain of her past, because she came to experienced me as an accepting person. Through our non-shaming connection, Vickie became more accepting of her own self and realized her sexuality was normal and natural, not something to be censored or condemned.

We can only heal what we feel. In Vickie's case, she experienced anger, fear, grief, and hurt as she unraveled the shame behind her eating disorder. The pain of recovery is like peeling the layers of an onion—tears and all!

It is only by getting in touch with our most authentic and genuine self and through honest sharing with others that we begin to move away from the despair caused by our inner sense of shame. In the past we sought relief through food, but it left us defeated and alone. Now we have other choices. Isolation with pastry needs to be replaced by intimacy with people.

Food for Thought Exercises

There is a saying, "We are as sick as our secrets." It is only when we share our deepest self that it is possible to heal a shame-based eating disorder.

Another saying, "We are all more human than not," reminds us that we are not as alone as we think. The range of human experiences—good, bad, and shameful—are shared to one degree or another by *all* of us.

1. How has shame played a role in the development of your eating problems?

2. What do you find most shameful about your eating problems ?

3. What is the most humiliating thing you have ever done with food?

4. How have you kept your eating problems a secret?

5. What do you consider most shameful about yourself?

6. What do you consider shameful about your family?

7. Were you shamed in your family for your eating, feelings, appearance, or crying?

8. Which of your emotional needs were most difficult for your family to deal with?

9. Which of your emotional needs are most difficult for *you* to deal with?

10. What is the most intimate thing you have ever revealed to another person?

11. What is the most intimate thing you have ever admitted about your eating problem?

CHAPTER 3

Sexuality and Self-Expression

When in doubt, tell the truth.
—Mark Twain

For many people with eating problems, the urge to eat compulsively, to purge, or to starve is often a substitute for love, intimacy, and sexuality. Fear and shame about expressing one's self sexually causes both men and women to avoid closeness—their relationship with food becomes the consuming passion instead.

Emotional eaters often find it safer to achieve intimacy by themselves with food than with a partner. Many women whom I have treated have expressed that putting food in one's mouth feels safer than sex through the vagina—*you* are in total control, *you* get to say how fast the food goes in, for how long, and you never have to hear from the food how *it* feels. Also, an intimate relationship with food can be easier than a sexual relationship in that you do not have to show your neediness to another human being. The food will never laugh or criticize you for how much you want or how you want it. You do not have to negotiate with the food, you do not have to ask it for favors or pleasures or a repeat performance. The food complies with you all the time.

No other physical act besides eating is so akin to sexual union. "The act of eating...consists of desire with salivation, the excitement of tasting and chewing, and the orgasmic contractions of swallowing, repeated again and again. While busy chewing and eating and thinking about food, [people] have little room in their psyches for sexual longings, for fears of intimacy, self-assertion, and dependence, or for anger and grief. They swallow and reach, swallow and reach."[1]

Fear of Expressing One's Self Sexually

Some people are afraid to express themselves sexually because they feel self conscious about whether their bodies measure up to the idealized image our culture fosters. Others struggle with deeper psychological issues which may be linked to traumatic events of the past, such as sexual abuse. Whenever people fear expressing sexual desire, though, they will seek another outlet for these powerful emotions. Turning to food is a common avenue.

Avoiding the Risk of Rejection

Many emotional eaters feel that asking to get one's sexual needs met is extremely risky. In her eating support group, Michelle described one of her midnight ice cream binges. She had wanted to make love to her husband and called out from the bedroom, "Are you coming to bed now?" When he answered that he still had work to do and would stay up for awhile, Michelle felt rejected and went straight to the Haagen Dazs. "You can always depend on ice cream," Michelle explained, "because the ice cream in my house never tells me that it has work to do!"

The group pointed out that Michelle's asking, "Are you coming to bed now?" might not be the best way to communicate her sexual desire. "But I thought if I asked him outright," she said, "it would have hurt even more if he had turned me down."

"You're right," the group answered. "There is a risk in asking. There is no guarantee he would respond to you in the way you wanted; but, by not asking directly, you are setting yourself up for a rejection which may not even be there."

"Well, I couldn't very well just say to him, 'I know you're busy but could you come to bed and make love anyway?' "

"Why not?" demanded the group. "You're entitled to ask. Asking certainly would have increased your chances of getting! And if he did say 'no,' does ice cream have to be your only solution?"

Through the group's support, Michelle realized for the first time how ashamed she felt in asking to have her sexual needs met. Having learned that initiating sex was the man's realm, she was uncomfortable taking the lead. However, by learning to use her mouth *to ask* instead of to eat, she began to break through the shame which had kept her unsatisfied, unchanged, and stuck in the ice cream.

This struggle affects men too. After their baby died a year ago, Eddie's wife seemed to lose interest in sex. In his attempt to be understanding, Eddie did not pressure Sheila to make love. Instead of discussing this with her, though, he turned to food as a substitute for sex. After some time, he also found himself fantasizing about having an affair with a woman at work. The guilt he felt about this sent him to the food even more, and in four months, he had gained 30 pounds. Without being entirely aware of it, Eddie was trying to make himself unattractive and thus prevent himself from having the affair.

To undo his "love affair" with the food, we worked to help Eddie express the shame he felt about still wanting sex despite his baby's death and his fear that his wife would be repelled by his desire. As he began speaking about these feelings with Sheila, she admitted to feeling guilty herself. She felt wrong for wanting sexual pleasure—or any other pleasure for that matter—as if that meant she were not grieving enough. By expressing their grief more openly with each other and discussing the guilt each was feeling, they felt closer in their shared pain. This gradually helped them experience a sense of renewed intimacy.

The Inability to Say No

Another fear expressed by emotional eaters is that if they lose weight and become more attractive to others, they might not be able to say "no" to unwanted advances and would regret their behavior afterwards.

Phyllis described her predicament: "When I lose weight, I love buying tight pants and showing off my body. If men start to notice, though, I get worried about not being faithful to my husband."

I responded to her inadvertently with a Freudian slip, "Well, let's look at what happens to you when you love buying tight *problems*." Phyllis and I laughed at how accurate my slip had been. The truth is that many emotional eaters often do have trouble saying "no" to more than just food, and saying "no" in a sexual relationship can be especially difficult. However, Phyllis learned that she could control the amount of contact she had with other men by identifying for herself what she wanted or did not want. She also began to speak up and discuss her dissatisfactions with her husband.

Our mouths have a dual purpose: to speak up and "dish out" our preferences or to stuff down food and squelch ourselves.

Fear of Ridicule

Emotional eaters often secretly feel insatiable about all their appetites—whether for food, love, or sex. Concluding that their partner will be turned off by their "excessive" sexual demands, they hide the full brunt of their longings rather than risk being ridiculed.

Recent studies of female sexuality, such as the *Hite Report*,[2] have shown that women can feel desire for longer, more extended periods of time than men. In another study, *The Nature and Evolution of Female Sexuality*, Dr. Mary Jane Sherfey explains that "the more orgasms a woman has, the stronger they become; the more orgasms she has, the more she can have. The human female is sexually insatiable in the presence of the highest degree of sexual stimulation."[3]

Just because a woman may feel embarrassed asking for second helpings at the dinner table, does not mean she needs to feel embarrassed asking for second helpings at sex. Although sometimes difficult, asking for the sex you want can be an antidote to eating problems. Only *chocolate* kisses have calories!

"Asking for what I want sexually? Easier said than done," says Andrea ruefully. "I couldn't even tell my husband I hated his beloved folk music until after we were married let alone ask for sex. I heard someone refer to emotional eaters as 'people pleasers,' and I know that applies to me. But I have come to realize that if I feel like I'm only getting crumbs during sex, I better say something or else I'll be checking out the cookies in the middle of the night."

Shame about Body Size

Shame about feeling fat is also a barrier to pursuing sex with more freedom. A woman who is an emotional eater may have particular feelings of vulnerability about whether she is attractive enough to her lover, and this will affect how comfortable she feels in communicating her sexual needs. Frequently a woman projects her own critical inner voice onto her partner.

Nancy always preferred having sex when she could be on top. After she gained weight following the birth of their third child, she was embarrassed to be in that position because her husband, Jim, would then see her belly protruding even more. Not only did she hate her weight, but she was also punishing herself by taking away the one position that guaranteed her pleasure.

Despite much embarrassment, Nancy eventually brought her worry out in the open with Jim, who was completely taken by surprise. He admitted to actually *preferring* her at a heavier weight because he felt more enveloped and snuggled in the sex act. It was her own self criticism that she mistakenly projected onto him which kept her blocked from permitting herself full pleasure.

Weight Struggles as a Smoke Screen for Other Issues

Cindy had a different experience with her husband. After she began a women's support group for binge eating, her husband Josh started complaining about her weight, claiming that he no longer found her sexually attractive. Since Cindy had been a large woman for several years, she was confused by this new criticism.

Through her therapy group, Cindy began to realize that as her own self-esteem increased, she was making more demands on Josh and was less compliant. She was beginning to "throw her weight around," and Josh was threatened by this. The only way he could find to assert himself was to criticize her weight, but now that Cindy had stopped bingeing and was feeling better about herself, she was less defensive.

Finally she was able to ask Josh openly why he had become so critical of her body. He admitted he was afraid that if she became thinner, she would become more independent and not need him as much. From this point on, the focus between them shifted from a battle about her weight to Josh's insecurities about their relationship. Cindy's weight had become a smoke screen for Josh which helped him avoid facing his fear about losing her. By becoming aware of the dynamics in their relationship, Cindy found the strength to speak up, confront her husband, and avoid consoling herself with food.

Why Should I Have to Ask?

Emotional eaters, with their "people pleasing" tendencies, rarely feel deserving enough to ask for what they need. Fearful to express themselves directly, they hope their partners can read their mind.

Sharon complained that she was frequently massaging her lover's back and playing with her hair, but Marilyn never reciprocated.

"Have you asked her for what you want?" I asked.

"But she should know," Sharon protested, "if she really loved me and thought about my needs."

"Really?" I said. "Why should she? You're expecting her to read your mind as proof of her love for you!" By saying, "Marilyn should know," Sharon was avoiding her own responsibility to ask and take care of her own needs in the relationship. Then, after lovemaking, Sharon would grab for the Doritos to stuff down her resentment at Marilyn's "insensitivity."

At times we all wish that another person will magically know how to make us feel good without our having to ask for anything. There is even a chocolate brownie on the market that exemplifies this wish called "Magic Mommy." This endearing name hints at the promise that the brownie has the power to soothe and take away all our troubles. How seductive!

Sexuality and Anorexia

This connection between emotional eating and sexual difficulties is not just the domain of compulsive overeaters. Fearful of embracing an adult body and adult sexuality, anorexics cope with their anxiety by starving themselves and halting the passage of time by remaining a skinny child.

Leah was typical of anorexic girls who equate fat with being rounded, female, and sexual. She came from a strict Orthodox Jewish family where great pressure was placed on girls to marry young. The only girl among six brothers, she was mother's "little helper." As she moved into puberty, the family began pressuring her to look fashionable, pretty, and slim. She obeyed—and then some. If her parents wanted a thin daughter, she would show them just how thin she could get. At 15, Leah became anorexic.

While other girls were growing up, Leah was growing "down." Starving became her silent, angry protest against the pressure of family and community. She started "reducing" herself to a child who could not be expected to think of marriage or babies. The idea of becoming sexual with a man terrified her. Her mother's experience taught her that sex meant repeated pregnancies, and that meant being extremely overwhelmed.

In the course of family therapy, her parents began to see the pain behind their daughter's anorexia. Gradually they started easing the pressure on Leah to grow up so quickly. She was then able to slowly emerge from her role as "Sleeping Beauty" to a three-dimensional young woman with vitality and opinions of her own.

Sexuality and Bulimia

Bulimia can also be a sign of sexual problems. Many bulimics have described that bingeing, vomiting and laxative abuse provide a safe substitute for sex because the act leaves them feeling more in control than they otherwise feel in their relationships with others. Bingeing and purging are similar in many ways to orgasm—an urgent, frantic buildup followed by feelings of satiety, and the orgasmic, spasmodic release from vomiting or laxative abuse.

People also become bulimic because they want to rid themselves of uncomfortable sexual feelings which they are not able to "digest." At age seven, Lillian had been molested by her alcoholic father. When she got married, she would binge and make herself throw up before making love with her husband because she felt dirty and guilty for "giving in" to her sexual feelings.

As we tried to make sense of what was happening to her, it occurred to Lillian that purging was her way of trying to get her father out of her system and thus free herself to be more fully with her husband. It was as if her father's abuse had left her with a bad "taste" about sex, and her vomiting was her attempt at exorcism. As a little girl, she had not been able to control what went in and out of her body, but, as an adult, bulimia became her way to take control and be in charge. After much painful work, Lillian confronted her father's betrayal and experienced her deep grief and rage. By expelling these emotions in her therapy sessions through talking and tears, Lillian discovered an outlet of relief other than through bingeing and purging.

Sexual Abuse and Eating Disorders

Sadly, no book about eating disorders is complete without a discussion of sexual abuse. In my practice, 40 to 60 percent of the men and women who come for therapy for an eating problem have been molested.

"It was my father's best friend." "It was my father." "It was my brother." "It was my mother's boyfriend." "It was my mother."

"And so I starved myself." "And so I ate." "And so I got fat." "And so I started using laxatives."

What is the connection between being sexually abused and developing an eating disorder? The answer is guilt, shame, anesthesia, self-punishment, soothing, comfort, protection and rage.

The experience of sexual abuse can have many different impacts on the eating and body image of survivors. Sexual abuse violates the boundaries of self so dramatically that inner sensations of hunger, fatigue, or sexuality become difficult to identify. People who have been sexually abused may turn to food to relieve a wide range of different tension states that have nothing to do with hunger, because they are confused and uncertain about their inner perceptions.

Survivors of sexual abuse often work to make themselves very fat or very thin in an attempt to render themselves unattractive, and in this way, try to de-sexualize themselves in the hopes of being more protected from sexual advances. Many survivors obsessively diet, starve, or purge to make their bodies "perfect." Having a perfect body is their attempt to feel more powerful, invulnerable, and in control, so as not to re-experience the powerlessness they felt as children. Some large men and women survivors are actually fearful of losing weight which might leave them feeling smaller and childlike, ushering in memories that are difficult to cope with.

Sexual Abuse and Secrecy

Sexual abuse and emotional eating both have one element in common. It is secrecy. Many eating disorder patients feel guilty about the sexual abuse in their childhoods, believing they could have prevented it but chose not to because of some defect in themselves. So they push their secret underground, and then distract and anesthetize themselves by emotional eating.

In most cases, children do not tell about their abuse because they did not realize at the time that anything wrong was happening. Those who are dependent on the abuser cannot risk upsetting the status quo. Often, children keep the abuse secret out of fear they will not be believed or because they were threatened or bribed to keep silent.

There are many nuances to sexual abuse beyond overt touching. One father repeatedly bragged to his daughter about the size of his testicles and how he needed special large underwear to accommodate them. Another patient reported how her father and brother would forcefully hold her down and tickle her all over until she was gasping for breath.

The Fear of Remembering

Every time Peggy became intimate with her boyfriend, she would stand over the kitchen sink gorging for the rest of the night, feeling scared, little and vulnerable. Peggy knew she had been sexually abused as a little girl, and she sensed there was a connection between this and her compulsive eating. Although she made many earnest attempts to remember, she could not get a clear memory— and so she continued to eat.

Shortly into her therapy, Peggy had the following dream: "I was sitting on my bed fishing. I had made a hole in the bed like the Alaskans do when they break through the ice to catch fish. Try as I might, I could not catch anything. Then I realized my fishing line had no hook!"

This dream helped us realize even more profoundly that Peggy, in her deepest self, was terrified to "hook" her memories. Although she was fishing for memories, and it was indeed like pushing through frozen layers of ice, she had neglected to add a hook to her line. At a subconscious level, she did not *want* to remember. In order not to feel her pain, Peggy truly wished the memory of her abuser to be "the big fish that got away."

Peggy's dream brought her to a crossroads in her recovery because she recognized that she would not be able to stop overeating until this part of her life was explored. She decided to commit herself "hook, line, and sinker" to becoming more open to the full knowledge of her abuse.

One day Peggy came home from work and went into her bedroom to change her clothes. There was her teddy bear, propped up on her bed just as she had left him that morning. His little legs were splayed open, and Peggy had a violent wish to ram her fingers up inside between the bear's legs. Then the dam of her blocked memories broke and she remembered vividly for the first time her father's drying her off after bath time and inserting his fingers harshly and repeatedly into Peggy's vagina. This flood of memories ushered in yet another period of out-of-control eating for Peggy, as she once again tried to block out the unbearable pain. Over a period of time, however, she shared her memories and her shame in our therapy sessions, and was able to face this agonizing betrayal and no longer needed food to protect her.

Post Traumatic Stress Disorder

People with eating problems often suffer from symptoms of post traumatic stress disorder without realizing its origins lie in sexual abuse. Post traumatic stress is sometimes characterized by depression, feeling chronically "dead" inside, recurrent anxiety or nightmares, or feeling constantly and painfully vigilant to one's surroundings. Some victims of post traumatic stress also engage in self-destructive behavior by forming repetitive abusive relationships, losing themselves to drugs, alcohol, promiscuity, or even self-mutilation.

Of course, none of these symptoms is absolute confirmation of abuse, but they are strong indicators of past sexual trauma. This is especially true if a person identifies several of these symptoms, since post traumatic stress disorder is usually a constellation of more than one indicator. Connecting these symptoms to an actual event of sexual abuse can be a validating experience because then symptoms of inner turmoil begin to make sense.

Healing from Sexual Abuse

What can you do to heal from sexual abuse? The first step is to recount your experience to someone you trust, someone with whom you can let yourself feel the brunt of your pain and rage. Since the experience of sexual abuse is about being out of control, you need to be in a protected setting where your feelings can reemerge and let loose. Releasing pain and guilt is not an intellectual experience, but something that comes from deep within. This can be a difficult step because exposing your emotions can feel like a reenactment of the original trauma.

Although there is more media coverage than ever before about the prevalence of sexual abuse, this does not relieve the shame that many people feel over it. If you have been a victim of incest, facing the abuse means facing not only the shame that you come from the kind of family where abuse is perpetrated, but also that no one in your family protected you. Additionally, men who have been sexually abused as children, either by a male relative or by their mother, have distinct shame issues related to feelings of passivity and weakness.

Sometimes eating disorder patients feel enormous guilt for having enjoyed the sexual contact with their abuser. Binge eating, purging or starving then becomes their ongoing self-induced punishment. When we scratch the surface of the lives of these children, though, we discover that sexual abuse may have been the only real affection or caring they received. A child who is lonely or starved for affection may revel in the attention, even if it is abuse. But the truth is that children are never the seducers—they are always the victims. The only thing a child is guilty of is the innocent wish to be loved.

Confronting your shame, releasing your pain, and experiencing rage and guilt are part of the process of reclaiming your inner self as well as your sexual self. The need to detour your feelings through destructive eating will subside when you are able to grieve for the little child who was betrayed.

Lately much has been written about "false memory syndrome" in which a person "remembers" sexual abuse that never occurred. This, indeed, can happen in certain vulnerable people. Therefore it is crucial that you not work with a therapist who "leads" you to a false memory of the experience. Memories of the abuse, if present, should evolve over the course of therapy rather than being planted in your head for you to "try on for size." If you suspect that something may have happened to you, trust your perception and let your inner "knowing" be your guide.

Declaring Peace with
Sexuality and Emotional Eating

Each of the people we discussed in the first part of this chapter had one thing in common—they developed a problematic relationship with food as a way of short-circuiting what they really need to be communicating to their partners. By turning to food, they were momentarily appeased, but were left unfulfilled in the long run because nothing had really changed in their relationships. Mustering the courage to ask directly for sex meant putting themselves in a vulnerable position, but to avoid doing so meant betraying their true need for intimacy.

Michelle of the midnight ice cream binges discovered that with humor, she could say a lot more to her husband than she ever dared to before. The next time around she called out to him, "Honey, either you come make love with me now or you'll have to go out and buy me some chocolate chip ice cream to take your place in bed." He decided to head for bed! Sharon was able to kid with Marilyn, "If you don't give *me* a massage treatment tonight, I'm calling up your mother to complain about *you*!" And Nancy, who worried that her husband would find her tummy too large, developed a little code language to help her laugh away her concern. "How about getting together for a belly laugh?" she would inquire.

The more we feel our sexual needs are legitimate, the easier it is to ask. We may not always get, but we have the right to ask. Sexual intimacy is the opposite of emotional eating. It is about surrendering, relaxing, sharing and letting go, while emotional eating is about controlling, rigidity, fear, and isolation. No amount of cookies, dieting, throwing up, or starving can satisfy sexual longings. In order to heal an eating problem, we need to reconnect our physical hunger with our stomachs and reconnect our sexual hunger with the appropriate organs!

Food for Thought Exercises

Many stages mark our transition from childhood to sexual adulthood. How we negotiate each of the stages will determine whether we exult in our sexuality or retreat behind the familiarity of food. See if you can pinpoint where in your sexual development the problem of emotional eating began for you.

Identifying the Stage: Think about how you negotiated each of these sexual turning points:

1. How did your parents, teachers, and religion explain sex to you? What were their attitudes towards sex and your developing sexuality?

2. If you are a woman, what were you told about menstruation? How did you feel when you got your period? If you are a man, what were you told about erections and ejaculation? What were you told about the opposite sex, and how did it make you feel?

3. Did you feel at ease exploring your body? Did you enjoy your sexual fantasies or feel uncomfortable with them?

4. Was your first sexual experience loving and tender or forced and painful?

5. Have you had homosexual experiences, and how has that influenced you?

6. Did you have any experiences of being sexually abused? How did you handle them? How do you feel it is affecting you now?

7. How was the role of wife and mother conveyed in your family? Did you feel that women were important and could be powerful?

8. What was the role of husband and father like in your family? Did you feel that men were important and could be powerful? Could they be tender and nurturing?

Where Are You Stuck?

There is a continuum of sexual expression. Identifying where along this continuum you divert yourself with food can help pinpoint what you need to work on.

1. Desire
2. Arousal
3. Initiation with your partner
4. Communicating your sexual needs
5. Orgasm
6. Shared intimacy

Working Toward the Resolution

1. If you had been your own mother, how would you have done things differently regarding your sexual education? If you had been your own father?

2. How would you raise your own child to avoid the pitfalls you may have experienced sexually?

3. What attitudes, advice, guidance would you like to be given today that would be healing to you?

CHAPTER 4

Anger and Assertiveness

She must learn again to speak
starting with I
starting with We
starting as the infant does
with her own true hunger
and pleasure and rage.
—Marge Piercy

Recently, in a neighborhood restaurant, I watched a mother and father eating dinner with their obese daughter who was wolfing down massive amounts of steak and potatoes, followed by pie with ice cream and whipped cream. As the young woman continued to eat voraciously, her parents began to squirm in their seats and look around the restaurant, almost apologetically.

I began to think about the power this daughter was wielding. Her size as well as her noisy display of eating seemed to be a reproachful accusation aimed at her family. Although she herself was probably in pain about her size, she appeared to be using her body to make a hostile statement to her parents which perhaps she was not able to make directly.

Anger and Eating

In my psychotherapy practice, I have witnessed time and time again the central role that unexpressed emotions, particularly anger, jealousy, hate, and rage, can play in creating and maintaining an eating problem. The pressure of keeping these feelings inside often becomes too great, and an emotional eater will recruit her own body to discharge them. Bingeing, purging, starving, and even obsessing about diets are all indirect ways of finding some relief from the pressure of unexpressed feelings—temporary though the relief may be.

Food is the safest, most available, abundant, and legal substance in the world for changing mood. It can "help" people: deny or distract themselves from angry feelings, anesthetize and numb hostile thoughts, vent feelings of rage through biting, chewing, purging, and starving, or postpone having to face the pain of deep inner conflict.

Anger is one of the most compelling of human emotions; there is an almost primitive connection between deep feelings of anger and hunger, biting, and chewing. The English language is replete with expressions that reveal this intrinsic connection:

"I couldn't stomach that situation."

"She's eaten up with envy."

"I wanted to bite his head off."

"I'm feeling fed up with how you're treating me."

"She swallowed her feelings of fury."

"She was enjoying the sweet taste of revenge."

"Her husband chewed her out."

"He's such a crumb."

"I have a bone to pick with you."

"Go eat your heart out!"

Even cooking terms illustrate food and anger connections.

"He was simmering with anger."

"She was at the boiling point with her husband."

"They were steaming mad at the landlord."

"He's so angry—he walks around like a pressure cooker."

"She's stewing about not getting the promotion."

"My supervisor made mincemeat out of me with his remarks."

"That speaker got such a roasting."

Anger Turned Inward Creates Eating Disorders

The connection between anger and eating disorders was brought home to me in an unusual way. I was in a comedy club one Saturday night listening to a comedian tell eating disorder jokes. The comedian said, "My mother was always a *blame*rexic—she keeps sticking her finger down *everyone else's* throat."[1] It occurred to me that if a bulimic were to redirect her finger from down her own throat, she would be pointing accusingly at someone else; but being too fearful of expressing her anger so directly, she chooses to hurt her own body instead.

Although this example described a bulimic, I began to appreciate the relevance this principle had for compulsive eaters and anorexics, as well. Over a period of time, unexpressed anger turns against the self, and the emotional eater will recruit her body to discharge her rage. The process goes something like this: "I am furious with you but I am afraid to tell you. So I will binge, vomit, or starve myself to get some of the hate I feel towards you out of my system."

In addition to feeling the pressure from such strong emotions, the emotional eater feels ashamed for harboring hateful feelings in the first place. Hate makes us feel like bad people. It is ugly. It makes us feel guilty. And this guilt can lead to further self-punishment. Eating disorders are all self-destructive behaviors; they are ways of attempting to "digest" our hostility.

Anger and the Overeater

Terry weighed over 400 pounds when she came to me for help at age 40. She was filled with self-hate and was tortured by how ugly and bad she thought she was. Terry was also stricken with remorse for having "failed" her mother, who had died two months earlier.

As we worked together on both her feelings of mourning and her gorging problem, we began to realize that not only did Terry believe that she had not been a good enough daughter, but she also felt abandoned by her mother. Mrs. Green had had several nervous breakdowns, was often too frightened to leave the house, and regularly left Terry in the care of her strict, cold grandmother.

Rather than expressing her animosity towards her mother, Terry felt guilty for even feeling that way. She turned the anger against herself, allowing it to "eat her up alive." Terry's train of thought went something like this: "I am angry. ➡ I should not feel that way. ➡ I am bad for having these thoughts. ➡ Where is the food to drown this all out?" Indeed, Terry was drowning in food, but she was also drowning in sorrow and fury for the little girl inside her who had never been nurtured enough. Terry was using food to "mother" herself and to stuff down her rage at feeling deprived.

Anger and the Bulimic

For the bulimic, both the binge and the purge can be ways to express anger. (This is not to deny that bingeing can also provide comfort and soothing.) The binge is a biting, chewing, devouring, aggressive kind of behavior. The purge—expelling the food through vomiting, laxative abuse, or driven exercise—is an attempt to purify one's self of these "bad" feelings. As is the case with compulsive overeaters, it is also a way of punishing one's self for having had these hostile feelings in the first place.

Barbara, a bulimic teenager, would binge and vomit to get attention from her mother, who only seemed to show concern when Barbara was heard vomiting loudly in the bathroom. "I sacrifice myself to piss my mother off," Barbara explained sarcastically. She was using her body and her bulimia to get back at her mother for neglecting her, but the physical pain of vomiting was *also* self-punishment for being so angry.

Anger and the Anorexic

Anorexia can be viewed as a way of trying to starve or "kill off" in fantasy someone in a patient's life with whom she is enraged—often a parent. Most often the anorexic's normal need for nurturing from her family has not been met. Over a period of time she begins to feel more and more abandoned and becomes suspicious of all nurturing—food included. Incapable of discharging her hostility directly, the anorexic unconsciously initiates a process of slow suicide. Her starvation becomes an aggressive act to punish the parent and to punish herself for harboring feelings of rage.

Debbie, a 22-year-old anorexic woman, felt that her wishes, her preferences, even her very identity were never respected by her family. "I was born a tomboy," Debbie explained, "but my parents insisted I wear dresses, curl my hair, and take ballet lessons. I hated all those girlie things, and I hated *them* for coercing me. Their control even extended to my eating. If I didn't like what we were having for dinner, they would force me to sit at the table until I cleaned every morsel on my plate. One night everyone went to bed leaving me at the table to finish my meal. I wouldn't. The more they escalated their demands, the more I refused to do what they wanted. Until I was hospitalized last spring, I was on a full blown hunger strike against them. Nobody was going to make me do anything I didn't want to."

Relationships and Anger

Issues of anger can be explosive in a relationship, and so we are often afraid to bring them out in the open. Avoiding these issues, however, can lead to a breakdown in communication between people and a retreat to or away from food.

Emotional eating has been called a disease of isolation because sometimes it is easier to be intimate with food than with people. Food never gets us angry, never disappoints, ridicules or breaks promises; but, in truth, there is no chocolate chip cookie in the world that can solve our relationship problems and our need for intimate connection.

Anger and Women

Expressing anger and asserting one's self are difficult areas for women in general, and for emotional eaters in particular. Our society emphasizes that women should behave in certain ways: "Be nice. If you don't have anything nice to say, don't say anything. Put others first. Don't make waves. Be lady-like." A woman who does express anger or conflict is labeled selfish, pushy, domineering, castrating, bitchy, or she is told, "you must be having your period."

A patient of mine, Greta, found herself gorging on Twinkies whenever she had to confront her husband about an issue that angered her. In one particular therapy session, she remembered a wooden sign that had hung in her father's study when she was a child. It portrayed an old fashioned woman with her head chopped off, and was titled, "The Silent Woman." As Greta ruefully revealed, this was definitely the message she received from her father early on—"*Women* should be seen and not heard!" So, she detoured her anger by eating—her way to "hold her tongue."

Anger and Fear

Fear also keeps anger stuck inside us. It can be scary to express anger directly, especially if we feel dependent on the person with whom we are angry. We all struggle with the prohibition, "Don't bite the hand that feeds you." The fear, of course, is that to bite the feeding hand is to lose it. Fear of abandonment or rejection keeps our mouths shut. No one wants to rupture a connection with someone they care about and need. In *The Struggle for Intimacy*, Janet Woititz discusses frequent misconceptions and fears about anger:

"If I'm angry with you, I don't love you."

"If you are angry with me, you don't love me."

"Since I do love you, then I can't allow myself to be angry."

"If you really love me, you will not be angry at me either."[2]

People who have been victims of physical abuse as children are particularly fearful of anger. They mistakenly believe that *any* expression of anger on their part will lead them to the same violent, out-of-control behavior they experienced from their parents. These people need to learn that there are many nuances of anger—from feeling vexed, piqued, turned off, cross, irritated, annoyed, frustrated, resentful, offended, bitter, indignant, insulted, and peeved, to furious, hateful, wrathful, and murderous.

When we cannot appreciate these different degrees or "gray areas" of anger, we are left with only black-or-white thinking. Fearful that any expression of anger would immediately turn her into an explosive, terrifying volcano, an anorexic patient explained, "I could only be angry at my mother if she were a bad person. My mother is not a bad person. Therefore I must not be angry at my mother."[3] This faulty "logic" was her way of talking herself out of being angry because she was so terrified of this feeling.

Anger and Guilt

We feel guilt over harboring mean and hostile thoughts toward others, especially if we also love them. Randy, a 35-year-old woman struggling with laxative bulimia, secretly hoped her best friend's expected promotion would not come through. Randy had recently had a setback on her own job and was jealous and angry that Claudia was doing better. Her guilt over her own angry wish that Claudia fail sent her into a frenzy of bingeing and laxative abuse. "I'm such a 'shitty' person for feeling this way," she said, and her laxative abuse was her attempt to evacuate these bad feelings.

Randy needed to learn that *feelings are not facts*. There is a world of difference between thought and action. Whatever she may think in the privacy of her head is permissible, understandable, and human. Her angry, jealous thought was just that—an angry, jealous thought. It was not the same as sending Claudia's boss an anonymous letter as to why she should not get the promotion!

The Value of Anger

"Anger is a signal, and one worth listening to. Our anger may be a message that we are being hurt, that our rights are being violated, that our needs or wants are not being adequately met. Our anger may tell us that we are not addressing an important emotional issue in our lives, or that too much of our self... is being compromised in a relationship. Just as physical pain tells us to take our hand off the hot stove, the pain of our anger preserves the very integrity of our self. Our anger can motivate us to say "no" to the ways in which we are defined by others and "yes" to the dictates of our inner self."[4]

Anger can be a catalyst for change in intimate relationships, a fuel that we can harness to help express ourselves. Honestly asserting our feelings can actually deepen intimacy. Loving someone and being angry at them are not mutually exclusive. It is only when we stifle our animosity and use food to detour around it, that we weaken its positive power and rob ourselves of its healing abilities. Many people who describe feeling numb or dead inside are actually working overtime to hold back angry, frightening feelings. The psychoanalyst, Otto Kernberg, wrote that it is often our failure to acknowledge our aggression which "transforms a deep love relation into... one that lacks the very essence of love."[5]

From the beginning of his marriage, Robert would dutifully visit his elderly father in the nursing home every Sunday, while Glenda stayed home with their baby feeling lonely and resentful. When their second child was born, Glenda was stuck at home even more of the time, and she was furious at Robert for leaving her. She did not express this anger, though, and rather than boil with rage, she boiled the water to binge on pasta.

Eventually, with the help of her eating support group, Glenda confronted Robert with how mad and rejected she felt. Her angry outburst then spurred Robert to vent his own unexpressed anger and resentment at having to trudge to the nursing home every week. He also shared with her some of the guilty feelings he felt toward his father. Glenda had never known how burdened Robert felt, but assumed that he had simply not cared that much about leaving her home alone. She now understood what it was like to be in his shoes.

It was only through expressing her anger that the door was opened for both Glenda and Robert to discuss solutions that could work for them. Glenda's open and honest communication was the tool that led the way toward deepening the intimacy in their marriage. As Glenda felt more understood, the call of the bingeing diminished and eventually faded away.

Expressing Anger

Cultivating your ability to say "no" when that is your preference is to increase your ability to say "no" to unwanted bingeing, purging, or starving, as well. Learning to say "no" is like exercising a muscle that gets stronger with practice.

Sandra described this aptly in her support group: "For me, food is a 'yes drug.' When I feel compelled to say 'yes' even though I don't really want to, I overeat to help me keep my mouth shut. In so many of my relationships, I sacrifice myself to keep the peace. But when I finally risk saying 'no' to another person, I no longer need the food to do the talking for me."

Sandra's story points out how our mouths can be used in two different ways: to eat, which can be a way of stuffing down our emotions, or to verbalize and release our hurts and anger.

There are times, though, when we cannot express our anger directly. If the person we are angry at has died or is in a position of power and can hurt us, or if we sense that our rage is too overwhelming, we must find another outlet. The essential ingredient, though, is to express ourselves— to a friend, to a support group, through imaginative fantasies, or through writing. The key is to find another avenue of release for the consuming urge to eat, purge or starve.

Bert wrote the following letter to his father who had been dead five years:

Dear Dad,

    I never got a chance to tell you how your drinking hurt me and how scared I was of you when I was growing up. I realize now that my bingeing and throwing up had a lot to do with swallowing my anger and fear, and I don't want to hurt myself anymore in that way. So I need to tell you I have hated you for cheating me of your love and guidance. I realize there are also many things I love about you, and perhaps I'll write you another letter telling you what they are. But for right now, I just need to give myself the chance to say I am angry with you and I wish you could have been different.

Your son,
Bert

A Remedy for Emotional Eating: A Separate Self, A Connected Self

Walt Whitman declared, "I celebrate myself, I sing myself." When we value, approve, and enjoy the entire range of our feelings and thoughts, anger does not feel so scary or destructive. Developing a strong *separate* sense of self, with clear boundaries and preferences, helps us stand our ground without wanting to hurt the people who make us angry. If we do want to hurt them, we can allow the fantasy without having to punish ourselves with eating problems.

To be a strong and independent self, however, is like clapping with one hand. Connecting with others and cultivating intimacy is equally necessary as an antidote for emotional eating. This intimacy requires learning to speak the truth with another person—angry feelings and all. Expressing ourselves authentically in a relationship— our fears, our hopes, our sexual feelings, and our anger— may be an ongoing struggle, but it is only when we share our real and vital selves that love becomes possible and food loses its power over us.

Food for Thought Exercises

Bingeing, purging, or limiting food intake can all be ways to sidestep anger. This assignment is to help you answer the questions, "What was eating me when I ate (or starved) and what stopped me from being more direct?"

Using a specific experience in which you used food to bypass your anger, examine:

1. At whom was your anger directed?

2. What did you want to say or do?

3. What did you actually say or do?

4. What were your fears about directly saying what you thought?

5. How did your eating problem "express" your anger?

6. Are you able to forgive yourself for harboring these angry thoughts?

CHAPTER 5

Overcoming the Fear of Success

*Fasten your seatbelts.
It's going to be a bumpy ride.*
—Bette Davis in *All About Eve*,
script by Joseph Mankiewicz

Our culture teaches us that the thinner we are, the better. Today's media bombards us with the message that thin equals sexy, young, successful, and happy. People often believe, "If only I were thin, my whole life would be happier."

A *Glamour Magazine* survey of 33,000 women revealed that 75 percent felt "too fat," although only one-quarter of these women were actually considered overweight by insurance table standards.

The New York Times has reported widespread abuse of diet pills among nine- and ten-year-old girls who are terrified of being fat.

Even a recent salami advertisement boasted their salami was leaner than the woman in their ad—and she was 79 percent fat-free!

What is Success?

Ironically, the quest for the "perfect" body—and the feelings of success that are reported to go with it—can backfire. The truth is that many people who are able to reach their goal weight continue to harbor deep feelings of hatred for their bodies. Even the emaciated anorexic can still feel fat and be "filled" with self-loathing. "Just as food never satisfied them, never gave them what they *really* wanted, so they are now dissatisfied with their new slim figure and disappointed in what it has achieved for them," says Hilde Bruch, a pioneer in the field of eating disorders, who coined the term "Thin/Fat" people to describe those who are no longer fat, but who continue to agonize about their weight. [1]

In other words, becoming thin might change a person's outer appearance, but it cannot guarantee that ingrained feelings of low self-esteem or inadequacy will vanish. Conversely, remaining large does not mean a person has failed to resolve an emotional eating problem. A large body is not necessarily an indication that someone is an emotional eater. Genetics, heredity, metabolism—factors over which we have no control or even a complete understanding—all contribute to pre-determining our natural size.

Successfully declaring peace with emotional eating, then, has little to do with thinness or fatness—it has to do with our *inner* state of mind. It means learning that food is not our enemy, that food was put on this earth to give us pleasure and to satisfy our hunger. True healing means learning other nourishing ways of comforting and soothing ourselves besides eating, and it means learning to feel at home in our bodies, treating them as a friendly ally rather than an object to be yelled at or criticized.

The Fear-of-Success Syndrome

With almost every patient I have treated for eating problems, I have discovered one obstacle which invariably raises its head. It appears most often just as a person begins to exert some control over his or her eating. It is what I call the "Fear-of-Success Syndrome."

Freud describes in his paper, "Those Wrecked by Success," that when some people attain a long cherished wish, they will fall ill because they cannot tolerate their wish coming true. Many emotional eaters have convinced themselves, in their conscious minds, that they are striving to resolve their destructive food thoughts and behaviors, but an unconscious part of them remains determined not to succeed.

The two main aspects of the Fear-of-Success Syndrome are fears of change and loss, and the need to sabotage ourselves.

Fears of Change and Loss

Human beings often experience any change, even change for the better, as a loss. Fears of change and loss come in many forms. Let's explore some of them.

Losing a Sense of Identity

Most emotional eaters spend a substantial amount of their thoughts and energy worrying about eating and weight—what they just ate, what they should have eaten instead, what they will eat tomorrow to make up for it. These thoughts and worries become second nature and in this way, provide a sense of identity and security. After all, to a great extent, we are what we think about.

Denise, who began therapy weighing over 300 pounds, is a case in point. She had lost 100 pounds the previous year, but had gained it all back and more. She felt helpless, frustrated, and in despair.

Denise came from a very religious family. When she broke away from their strict teachings, her wish to lose weight became her new "religion," but with unexpected results. "As I got thinner, I also became depressed," Denise revealed. "I had a feeling of loss that was similar to what I felt when I moved away from my family and the religious beliefs I grew up with. If I couldn't worry about losing, gaining, dieting, and calories, what would give my life meaning? Telling myself I am fat and ugly has been like a daily mantra for me! What am I going to replace that with? If I give up my obsession with food and weight, I worry about feeling empty inside and without purpose."

This identity crisis also occurs in patients who come for therapy following a dramatic weight loss due to a fast. Marla had lost 110 pounds this way, but found herself bingeing again. She came for help in a state of terror, explaining that at her new thin weight, she no longer knew who she was. "I feel like a stranger in a strange land. I now have to learn how to navigate my body through life at this new weight—how to walk down the street, how much space I need to sit on a bus. It scares me. All of this is so new. I don't even know what style clothes I like or what size I should wear. Even my face looks unfamiliar."

Both Denise and Marla found themselves in a period of transition and mourning that many emotional eaters experience when their obsession is no longer at the forefront. The ability to tolerate this transition period and work through it is a vital key to sustained recovery. In addition, their stories illustrate an issue central to recovery: How to give one's life meaning and structure beyond the consuming security blanket of food, weight and dieting?

Losing the Status Quo in Relationships

Sometimes, weight is an integral factor in the balance of power, trust, and dependency in relationships. Removing that ingredient means having to find new ways of relating to others.

Peter's wife and daughter badgered him constantly about losing weight. In despair, they finally joined a family support group which helped them realize the futility of trying to control Peter's behavior. As they backed off from criticizing him, Peter discovered how much he missed their complaining about his weight! Their attention had made him feel cared for and special. He said, "It was similar to my family of origin where my mother repeatedly berated my father to stop drinking. I never realized that I interpreted her reprimands as a way of showing my father love and attention. I'm beginning to see that my need to be scolded by my wife and daughter is some kind of misguided attempt to get their affection. Unfortunately, what it really is doing is eroding their respect for me."

Changing the status quo of intimate relationships is frightening and can be a threat for family members, as well. In *Fat is a Family Affair,* Dr. Judi Hollis discusses a study of husbands' reactions to their wives' weight loss:

> "These men worried that they would (1) lose a binge buddy; (2) lose the advantage of saying 'You fat slob, what do you know?' They anticipated not the joy of having an attractive spouse, but a fear that their wives' heightened self-image might destroy the relationship. She might have new options: divorce and infidelity. These men expressed more fear of loss than anticipated joy of success."[2]

Power struggles between husbands and wives about weight also affect the status quo. Imagine the stress and confusion of a wife whose husband says, "Honey, you really need to lose a couple of pounds." But if Honey starts losing those pounds, he suddenly becomes worried and brings her a box of chocolates to celebrate!

People with anorexia also acknowledge that their thinness gives them a special role in the family and that restoring their weight might mean losing that attention. My patient, Mary, confided, "I am an identical twin, and since I've gotten so thin no one mistakes me for Grace anymore. Before, my family was more worried about me than her and that gave me a sense of secret power. Now I'm realizing that getting attention by staying anorexic is a hollow victory—being special for being thin is not the same as being special for being me!"

Sometimes being successful feels like being disloyal to our family, and so we sacrifice ourselves to continue to belong. Betsy came from a family of obese parents and two obese brothers who shared an ongoing camaraderie about their weight. When Betsy went away to college, she was able to get more in touch with her own rhythm of eating and lost 20 pounds. But when she returned home for Thanksgiving, her family treated her as if she had deserted them. "Boy, look at her," they said. "College makes you think you're too good for us. We have two weeks to fatten you up again!"

Betsy was devastated by her family's disapproval and began to feel guilty about her change in size. She started to overeat to undo her achievement and "return to the fold." In therapy, though, she realized that regaining the weight was her way of trying to keep the relationship with her family intact. She also understood that her success—

whether it was enjoying her body more or achieving a college education—would entail some degree of growing beyond and apart from her family. As she slowly resolved this anxiety and guilt about separating from her family, she was able to get back on track with her new-found patterns of healthy eating.

Losing a Sense of Sexual Protection

When we don't know how to negotiate sexual advances, we can make our bodies very skinny or fat in order to feel more powerful and in control. Some anorexic girls starve themselves to eradicate their feminine curves; anorexic boys seek to diminish their muscular development in the hope of desexualizing themselves. Reducing one's body to that of a child is an attempt, in part, to ward off the fears and responsibilities of sexuality.

Those who make their bodies large through bingeing may also be trying to desexualize themselves. "The more space my body takes up, the more distance there is between you and me." To lose that "protection" can feel dangerous and scary.

In truth, becoming skinny or fat does not have the power to desexualize us. People of all sizes and shapes can be sexually active and satisfied. Real power lies in having choices and in developing our ability to express and act on those choices: learning to say, "yes" when we mean, "yes," learning to say, "no" when we mean, "no," and learning to say, "maybe" when we haven't quite decided.

Lorraine had been sexually abused by her uncle when she was ten. At age 19, she found herself in a sexual situation with a man from work and became terrified. She feared that this man would overpower her and that she would be left vulnerable, without any control over the situation. She began gaining weight, hoping that it would "shield" her from his advances.

In therapy, Lorraine and I worked together to help her relive and resolve the pain of her uncle's abuse. Gradually she began to separate her past experience from her present. She discovered that she *did* want to connect with this man, but in a manner that felt comfortable for her. So, Lorraine worked on developing the realm of "maybe," which included a degree of flirtation. Lorraine didn't necessarily want the "full course meal," but she wanted to try the "appetizer"—to laugh and banter and be playful. Flirting gave Lorraine another option besides retreating. It also enabled her to feel more in control of the contact and less dependent on her weight to protect her. In time, she even felt secure enough to taste the main course!

Losing Other Women's Approval

Fear of alienating other women and losing their support is an undercurrent for many women who begin to gain healthier bodies and feel more attractive. Being overweight, or even substantially underweight, intimates: "I am not a threat." "You don't have to worry about my being prettier than you or stealing all the attention." When a woman succeeds in feeling more in harmony with her body, she fears putting herself back in competition with other women.

Envy and competition are uncomfortable feelings for women to have for one another. Sometimes, having our girlfriends envy us validates our success, but it also brings with it the possibility that they will withdraw their affection and desert us. The question then arises, "How powerful or attractive can I become without causing my friends to reject me?"

In their book, *Between Women,* Luise Eichenbaum and Susie Orbach explain that "we can feel guilty for our strivings and seek punishment for them. The unconscious equation that fulfilling oneself, succeeding in one's career, or achieving a personally satisfying love relationship is a betrayal of another woman (mother) is extremely common. We can imagine or project onto one another disapproval and in this way we hold each other back."[3]

Of course, this is not a perfect world and there may be people in our lives who resent our freedom from obsession with food and weight. But the more we can tolerate their envy and let the problem be theirs and not ours, the more we will be able to hold onto our successes and not abandon ourselves by returning to emotional eating.

Naomi told her eating support group that whenever she felt more attractive, she became afraid that her girlfriends would desert her. Naomi's mother had been a fashion model and always needed to be the most beautiful woman in the family. The friends Naomi would bring home from school would say in surprise, *"That's* your mother?" impressed by Mrs. Fisher's glamour.

When Naomi began blossoming at age 13, her mother became quite critical of her. "I couldn't win," she said. "My mother was always prettier and sexier. There was room for only one attractive female in our house—she made that clear. For me, not bingeing anymore and getting to my natural weight brings back awful memories of my mother's competitiveness, and makes me think my girlfriends are going to hate me. In this group, though, the women are *not* my mother. They applaud my progress. They want me to succeed. This is very healing for me. Enjoying and nurturing my body doesn't have to lead to abandonment."

Losing Physical Protection

Some people may unwittingly want to be fat because of their fears about being physically vulnerable at a smaller size. Patients in my eating support groups have even expressed anxiety about losing weight because they connected thinness with the pain of watching a loved one become emaciated from cancer. As irrational as these thoughts may seem, they nevertheless can exert a powerful influence on our willingness to make peace with food and allow our bodies to reach their natural weight. These connections need to be uncovered and untangled so their power over us can be lessened.

Ruth: "When I was nine years old, a girl in my class fell between the subway cars and was killed. She had just lost over 50 pounds, and I kept thinking if she were still fat she wouldn't have been able to fall between those cars. This made an enormous impression on me, and I started to link my own weight loss with the fear that something terrible could happen to me, too."

Annette: "I was hit by a bicycle last week, and I remember thinking, 'It's a good thing I'm fat or I would have gotten really hurt.' "

Lois: "My father was fat all his life, and in the last two years the doctors convinced him to lose weight because his health was in jeopardy. He finally did lose 65 pounds, but died six months later from a stroke. I always felt that if he hadn't lost so much weight, he never would have died. It made me scared that could happen to me."

Losing the Power to Spite Someone

From the minute she was born, it seemed to Alice that her mother only wanted two things from her: that she be slim and get married to someone rich. But try as she might, Alice could not lose the extra 50 pounds her mother hated and only managed to meet down-and-out guys. "Since I was a little girl, my mother measured out my food and weighed me weekly. I hated scales. I hated measuring cups. I hated her! Whenever her back was turned, I would sneak candy and cookies. Keeping myself fat was perfect revenge, and even though I'm now 25, my mother is still trying to control my weight and marital status—and I'm still reacting!"

"What's pathetic about my story," Alice continued, "is that I'd really like to have normal eating habits and get married some day. But another part of me enjoys getting back at her more than getting my life together. I'm in such a bind!"

Alice knew that if she did lose weight, she would also lose a powerful weapon against her mother. Staying large is her way of communicating, "I'm going to be my own person, and you can't do anything about it!" This is reminiscent of the daughter in the motion picture, *Summer Wishes, Winter Dreams,* who yells at her mother, "Don't criticize me about my weight. It's the only thing that's mine, and you are not going to take that away from me!"

Only when Alice learns to separate her wishes and hopes for herself from the coercion and pressure she experiences from her mother, will she be able to permit herself to attain her natural weight. This means asserting herself directly rather than letting her body do the talking for her. Then, her decisions will come from within *her* and not from her mother. As a colleague of mine once said, "Maturity is doing something *even though* your mother wants it!"[4]

There is a group of patients who do not want to succeed in resolving their eating problems, because they have an investment in trying to spite the therapist. Their interest in robbing the therapist of the pleasure of helping them and being important to them is based on early issues of envy and competition with a parent. The wish to get even with parents who have been controlling or authoritative leads the patient, often unconsciously, to undermine his own progress in therapy.

Overcoming the Fears of Change and Loss

In her book, *Necessary Losses,* Judith Viorst reminds us that losses are a necessary and vital part of life that can spur us on to change and grow. "The road to human development is paved with renunciation. Throughout our life we grow by giving up. We give up some of our deepest attachments to others. We give up certain cherished parts of ourselves. We must confront all that we will never have and never will be. We grow by losing and leaving and letting go. We grow by changing and moving on."[5]

A powerful step toward sustaining progress is to recognize that our success may usher in anxiety about loss. People often backtrack because they are only dimly aware that giving up bingeing, purging, or starving can create its *own* stress that needs to be dealt with.

Lorraine, whose uncle had molested her when she was little, joined a group for incest survivors which encouraged and supported her to express her deep sense of betrayal, rage, and sadness. Lorraine's inner mechanism of saying "no" had been damaged as a child because of this experience with her uncle. She had lost her sense of having a separate self—one with the capacity to set limits, and this had carried over to her difficulty in setting limits with food. As she began expressing her rage, Lorraine felt more powerful and was able to reclaim her ability to say "no" both to food and to unwanted sexual advances. This enabled her, in the end, to say "yes" when that was her wish.

"Honey," on the other hand, whose husband celebrated her weight loss by presenting her with a box of chocolates, needed to face her disappointment and anger at him for trying to coerce her into living up to his image of how a wife should look. Rather than retreating back to the bonbons, Honey decided to confront her husband and put the *issue of her anger* on the table!

It takes courage to grow and succeed. This courage will help us stay on the path and will lead us from pain to empowerment. Growing pains got its name because sometimes growing hurts!

Self-Sabotage

In addition to fears of change and loss, many people fail to declare peace with emotional eating because of an unconscious need to sabotage themselves.

Anger Turned Inward

Patients often replay within themselves an angry, hateful relationship they once had as children with their mother or father. Instead of expressing their feelings directly, they punish themselves to make up for feeling hateful in the first place. This was the case with Carolyn, a 35-year-old woman who suffered from bulimia.

When Carolyn was a little girl, her mother seemed more interested in card games with her friends than in her daughter. When Carolyn tried to get some attention, she was banished to her room, or worse, her mother would simply give her the "silent treatment." Carolyn remembered wanting to cry and scream, but she was too afraid of losing her mother. Instead, she began acting out.

"One day, I remember feeling furious with my mother for not letting me take ballet lessons. That night I went up to my room and cut down the hem of my favorite dress to get back at her. I knew my mother hated to sew, and I knew this would upset her, but I never realized until I came to therapy that the reason I chose my *favorite* dress was to punish *myself* because I felt so guilty for being such an angry, hateful kid."

Carolyn first came to therapy because she was struggling to overcome violent bingeing and purging episodes. We began to see how this type of behavior was similar to her skirt-cutting as a child. In both cases, she was discharging a tremendous amount of bottled up rage and engaging in a form of self-sabotage. She was turning the anger she felt towards her mother against herself by hurting her body as an adult just as she damaged her skirt as a child. The battle between Carolyn and her mother now continued within Carolyn herself—a civil war.

In the book *Self-Realization and Self-Defeat,* Samuel Warner explains that self-defeat is a technique to achieve power over others and get indirect revenge. "All of us learn in childhood that we can 'get back' at others by defeating ourselves. It is an element of childhood's repertoire mechanisms for dealing with life. And thus the stage is set for the utilization of self-defeat as a way of venting unconscious resentment in life. Self-defeat is always self-and-*other* defeat."[6]

Guilt and Self-Sabotage

People do not feel entitled to success for other reasons, many of which relate to inner feelings of guilt. In his book, *Why People Fail,* Dr. Herb Strean describes the psychological meaning of failure and how, if we believe our success will make others suffer or if we feel that in becoming successful we have stolen happiness away from someone else, we will arrange to defeat ourselves so we do not have to feel guilty. If we surpass our rivals, we may view our accomplishments as provocative acts that hurt others, which then makes us feel obliged to undo our success.[7]

People do not feel entitled to success for many reasons:

"If it weren't for me, my parents wouldn't have gotten drunk (divorced, sick, fought so much, died, etc.)."

"My mother was never able to lose weight, and I don't want to make her look bad."

"I was sexually molested as a child and part of me enjoyed that attention."

"My sister was retarded. How can I feel good about still another accomplishment?"

Many patients who come to see me for therapy make great strides in improving their relationships and professional lives. When they are also able to declare peace with their eating problems, they often worry that they now, "Have it all." Unless this guilt is recognized and worked through, they will weaken their own progress as penance for the idea that they are hurting other people who are not as lucky as they are.

Overcoming Self-Sabotage

In *Compassion and Self-Hate*, Dr. Theodore Isaac Rubin speaks of compassion for one's self as the antidote to self-punishment and self-hate. Compassion is a state of forgiveness, of benevolence, of declaring peace with ourselves, which we can generate:[8]

- By accepting the fact that achieving success in our lives means, to some degree, abandoning the cocoon of our families.
- By accepting that we can love and hate someone all at the same time, and these feelings, although conflicting, are fully human and not worthy of self-punishment.
- By accepting that we can entertain all kinds of thoughts in the privacy of our heads from murder to adultery, but thinking these thoughts is not the same as acting on them and therefore not worthy of self-punishment.
- By accepting that putting our own needs first is not selfish but based on self-love and self-preservation. To be "people pleasers," on the other hand, is to ignore our own healthy self-interest.
- By accepting that the daily living of life is not a dress rehearsal for some future performance. The present moment is all we have, and we have a responsibility to make it the fullest and richest life we can.

To sum up the attitude needed for working out our fear of success: "Feel the fear and do it anyway!"

Food for Thought Exercises

Resolving an eating problem can arouse strong feelings of fear, especially when success involves so many intense changes. If you were living in harmony with your body and expressing your feelings without detouring them through dieting, bingeing, purging or starving:

1. How would your family life change? Your work life? Your friendships?

2. In what ways would these changes be negative or frightening?

3. In what ways would these changes be positive or exhilarating?

4. Are there any other "dangers" about declaring peace with your food and eating that could get in your way?

Each of the fears of change you discover needs to be tackled with a three-pronged approach:

1. Identifying and confronting the feelings of loss that emerge as you begin to succeed.

2. Finding an outlet of self-expression that can give meaning to your life outside of the consuming passion with weight and food.

3. Moving beyond the loss to new ways of empowering yourself either by joining a support group, entering therapy, or developing an inner spiritual life.

CHAPTER 6

Addiction
When You Are Powerless

Lead me to the rock which is higher than I.
—Psalms 61:2

The most humiliating experience I ever had with food occurred the year I lived in Spain. I tell this story because it was a turning point along my road to recovery.

I was living with a Spanish family while attending the University of Seville. At night, I would sneak food out of their cupboards when they were asleep as I had done back home with my own family. My favorite "sneak" was the cookies with the Virgin of the Macarena printed on the label. Eating stealthily, standing up in someone's kitchen thousands of miles from home would have been shameful enough in my own eyes, but one awful night, I realized the cookies had ants on them. I tried to brush the ants off while still devouring the cookies. The throes of the binge had me caught in its momentum. This is what I call addiction.

Addiction is when:

Your need for the gratification of the moment becomes more urgent than your rational self.

Your stomach and better judgment says, "Please. No!" and you eat anyway.

You lie to others about what you are eating and sneak food behind their backs.

You avoid socializing or going to work in order to binge, purge or starve.

You cannot stop eating compulsively, vomiting or starving despite your best efforts.

You are ashamed and humiliated by your eating but feel powerless to do anything to help yourself.

You use food—either by overeating, purging, or starving—to change your mood, lift your spirits, put yourself to sleep, or deep-freeze painful feelings.

At the time, I felt powerless over my relationship with food, and I began to explore the idea that I might have an addiction. Although I traveled down many paths to finally arrive at what works for me today, my connecting with the addiction approach to healing became the first step in my journey.

Physiological Illness/Psychological Obsession

Addiction is a complex *physiological illness* coupled with a *psychological obsession* which progresses over time. Food addiction is considered a disease by some who say that it cannot be cured but only arrested one day at a time.

Physiologically, food addicts need to consume increasingly large amounts of food to feel good. Usually the addict is drawn to foods high in sugar, fat, salt, or wheat products. Unlike normal eaters, food addicts have a very high tolerance for consuming large amounts of these foods and will experience withdrawal when they cannot get their food "fix." Symptoms of withdrawal may include crying spells, insomnia, irritability, difficulty concentrating, feelings of rage, depression, fatigue, and headaches. The withdrawal symptoms then set up further cravings for even more food.

Increasing evidence suggests food addicts may have a metabolic abnormality of their body chemistry which causes them to crave refined carbohydrates, such as sugar, in the same way that an alcoholic craves liquor. Carbohydrates cause the body to release the chemical serotonin, which is a natural calming agent that eases feelings of stress and tension. Bingeing then, is really an attempt at self-medication—a way of raising the body's serotonin level.

Starvation also produces a "kick" for people with anorexia because endorphins (the body's natural feel-good chemicals) are released by a lack of food. Compulsive exercise provides a similar "kick" as well. Thus we see that people may become "committed" to their addiction not because they lack willpower, but because of strong biochemical forces.

A food addict also develops an intense mental obsession with food—whether to eat or not eat, gain or lose weight, keep food in or purge it out, how much to exercise, how many calories to eat, how to best diet. This "consuming" preoccupation can interfere dramatically with day-to-day living, as well as drain one's energy from the pursuit of far more enriching life goals.

Progressive Stages

According to the addictions theory, the symptoms of eating disorders become increasingly life-damaging over time. For this reason, every food addict goes through progressive stages of decline.

In the case of a person with anorexia, the early stage of the disease is marked by a distorted body image in which she feels fat, despite being emaciated. She suffers from low self-esteem and deep anxiety about being in control of her life. (Since the majority of anorexics are female, I will use the female pronoun here.) In the middle stage, she hits on a perfect remedy for these feelings—a diet. Although she may not be able to control her life or the people around her, she can control her food and does so with a vengeance. The diet, however, begins to take on a life of its own as the anorexic continues to reduce the amount of food she eats. She loses at least 15 percent of her body weight, menstruation ceases, and she may begin compulsive exercising. In the last stage of the illness, she withdraws from family and friends, becomes more isolated and rigid in her behavior, and has difficulty concentrating. Unless she can recognize her need for help and can start to take steps toward recovery, she may die from malnutrition, cardiac arrest, or electrolyte imbalance.

People with bulimia follow a similar downhill course. Also believing that their self-worth depends on thinness, bulimics try to compensate for their perceived overeating by purging. In the first stage they may experiment with vomiting, laxatives, diuretics, or over-exercising. In the middle stage, bingeing and purging may take over to the extent that bulimics will resort to stealing and lying to satisfy their need for increasing amounts of food. They usually become distant from family and friends and sometimes abuse drugs, alcohol, laxatives, or diuretics. Symptoms include chronic sore throats from vomiting and gastrointestinal disorders from laxative abuse. Unless bulimic sufferers can recognize their need for help, they can die from rupture of the heart or esophagus, peritonitis, or, in extreme cases of deep despair and hopelessness, they may commit suicide. At the very least, they will lead lives of secrecy and escalating emotional and physical pain.

Compulsive eaters begin the course of their disease by gorging on food in order to assuage stressful or painful feelings. They then try various diets with only temporary success. In the middle stage of the disease, they become socially isolated because eating takes up increasing amounts of their time. Unless compulsive overeaters can break through their denial and recognize their need for help, they will become more dishonest with themselves and ashamed about socializing. Health problems such as heart disease, diabetes, hypertension, gastrointestinal disorders may develop in certain large people.

Recovery from Addiction—The OA Approach

Recovery for all addicted eaters begins when they recognize that their lives have become unmanageable and they are powerless over food. For the food addict, relief may come with a program such as Overeaters Anonymous.

OA is a self-help group of men and women which offers a rich resource of structure, support, and compassion for breaking out of the bondage of eating problems. It is one of the many ways to heal from struggles with food and eating.

In the meetings, people share their experience, strength, and hope with other members. This particular program is based on the format of Alcoholics Anonymous, which was founded in 1935 by two alcoholics who were struggling to remain sober and discovered that *reaching out to one another* for support was the crucial ingredient that sustained their sobriety.

The book *Alcoholics Anonymous*, affectionately known as *The Big Book*, explains the guiding principles of the Program. "The fact is," *The Big Book* says, "that most alcoholics have lost the power of choice in drink. Our so-called willpower becomes practically nonexistent. We are unable, at certain times, to bring into our consciousness with sufficient force the memory of the suffering and humiliation of even a week or a month ago. We are without defense against the first drink... There is a complete failure of the kind of defense that keeps one from putting his hand on a hot stove."[1] Many people with eating disorders can identify with these feelings.

It was with great trepidation that I crept into my first meeting of OA. I decided to go because a friend of mine who had joined was getting her compulsive eating under control and described feeling more inwardly peaceful. My jealousy, curiosity, and righteous skepticism prompted me to give it a try.

Another friend, Susan, had cautioned me, "They are a bunch of primitives." If anyone were to ask, I was prepared to say that I was a visitor looking to expand my knowledge base. I don't know whom I was planning to fool, since I'm sure I looked visibly terrified!

Actually, working at a mental health clinic had given me some idea of what Alcoholics Anonymous counselors were all about. They walked around carrying coffee cups that read, "One Day at a Time." If you asked them how they were, they'd say, "Clean and Sober, thank you" or

"Keeping it Simple. Just for Today." They were like a tribe that had acquired a limited number of slogans to be used interchangeably in any conversation, whether it was about politics, job stress, or the weather.

I stole out of my first meeting a half hour after I arrived. The following week I did the same. Much to my dismay I was becoming intrigued with the Program in spite of myself. Gradually I stayed and discovered that the "primitives" included people like me who felt out of control in their relationship with food.

Early on, I met Esther who became my sponsor. She explained that I was powerless over food, and it was making my life unmanageable. "But how do I go about losing weight?" I asked impatiently. "This isn't a diet club," she responded. "It's about being abstinent—following a daily food plan and working the Steps. The weight will take care of itself. The body nature gave you is what you are after."

Every day I called Esther and talked to her about my trials and tribulations with eating. This was exhilarating since I never had confessed to anyone what I did in secret with food. She taught me to make a commitment to her each morning about what I would eat that day, and I would then be relieved for the rest of that day from obsessing about that decision. She taught me to forgive myself if I had problems with food and overeating, and showed me that I was entitled to my own compassion no matter what I did.

I also began developing friendships with other people in the Program. Selena taught me that "an extra bite was just a bite," not an inevitable fall from grace. Sharon taught me that my lifestyle, in which I always managed to see the cloud in every silver lining, had contributed to my eating problem. She also taught me to meditate and let go of my need to control everything and everybody. With Rebecca I discussed matters of the heart that would have previously led me to overeating. I enjoyed being part of a group where people cared about being honest with themselves and with each other about what they did in the privacy of their kitchens. We laughed, cried, and confessed together. Isolating myself with food was replaced by warm, intimate sharing with other people.

OA became a turning point in my life because it broke through my false belief that I could stop bingeing and yo-yo dieting whenever I wanted. For the first time I felt I had a choice. I did not have to continue doing the same hurtful behavior to myself for the rest of my life.

A Three-Fold Approach

Overeaters Anonymous believes that eating problems are a three-fold disease: physical, emotional, and spiritual. The problem is emotional, the symptom is physical, the solution is spiritual.

The Program is comprised of three ingredients:
- The Steps
- The Meetings
- The Tools

The Steps

The Twelve Steps of OA, modeled on the Alcoholics Anonymous Twelve Steps, are the backbone of the Program. Only one step deals directly with food; the others address our relationship to ourselves, to others, and to a Higher Power.

Because the steps talk about God, many people believe that OA is a religious program and therefore not for them.

However, the Program emphasizes that each individual should choose a concept of a Higher Power that fits their understanding and belief system. This concept then becomes a strength they can turn to for guidance that is greater than their momentary desires and compulsions for food. Many people consider the collective strength of the OA group to be their Higher Power. Some believe that God refers to Good Orderly Direction. Others define the concept of God as their own true, inner voice—the part of themselves where their most honest and caring self resides. Sometimes OA-ers simply call God my "better judgment."

It has been said about alcohol addiction that, "To be defeated by the bottle and to know it is the first 'spiritual experience.' The myth of self-power is broken by the demonstration of a greater power."[2] When we think how we have made food our God—or the craving for thinness or the number on the scale—the idea of choosing a healthier concept to rely on for help and guidance becomes easier to understand.

The twelve steps of the Program are as follows:

1. We admitted we were powerless over food—that our lives had become unmanageable.

When the pain of eating, starving, purging, or chronic dieting becomes greater than the pain of not doing those behaviors, you are ready for this step. In his book *Compulsive Overeater*, Bill B. writes, "The willingness to accept the first step every day of our lives releases us from the bondage of ourselves."[3] Often we need to hit rock bottom before we realize that the battle to eat or not to eat has gotten the best of us. This step encourages us to stop fighting and surrender to the fact that willpower has never cured us of anything.

2. Came to believe that a Power greater than ourselves could restore us to sanity.

"I tried doing it alone and it didn't work," is the essence of this step. For the addict, no amount of promises, pleading, or penitence is going to break the bondage to emotional eating. "We have the *inability* to control our eating," says Bill B.

3. Made a decision to turn our will and our lives over to the care of God *as we understood Him.*

If we can let go of our need to control everything and everybody and become attuned to the inner voice of our better judgment, we can break food's compulsive grip on us.

4. Made a searching and fearless moral inventory of ourselves.

In our inventory, we list our resentments, angers, and the hurtful things we have done to others. This is not because we want to become altruistic Pollyannas, but because harboring these feelings has led to our consoling ourselves with food.

5. Admitted to God, to ourselves, and to another human being the exact nature of our wrongs.

This step provides a path to deal with our mistakes. We can alleviate our shame by admitting our character problems to ourselves, sharing them with another person and with our Higher Power.

6. Were entirely ready to have God remove all these defects of character.

To achieve this step, we "must become willing to live without the negative excitement of feeling bad" and be ready to let go of the aspects of our personality that have caused us to overeat, purge, or starve.

7. Humbly asked Him to remove our shortcomings.

This step is about humility. When I was in OA, the character defect that I most wanted to hold onto was my well-practiced gift of complaining. I agreed with the comedian Lily Tomlin that the reason God gave human beings the power of speech was so we would be able to complain! To let go of this outlet meant I would be robbed of my most important means of communicating! I had to ask for extra help with this. God helped me replace my negative tendencies with a more wry and humorous vision of life.

8. Made a list of all persons we had harmed, and became willing to make amends to them all.
and...
9. Made direct amends to such people wherever possible, except when to do so would injure them or others.

In these steps we try to confront our past mistakes, unburden ourselves of guilt, and earn back the self-esteem that may have been eclipsed by our emotional eating. The Program promises us, "We are going to know a new freedom and a new happiness. We will comprehend the word serenity and we will know peace. We will suddenly realize that God is doing for us what we could not do for ourselves."[4]

10. Continued to take personal inventory and when we were wrong, promptly admitted it.

In this step we practice the Program on a daily basis in all aspects of our lives. We need to constantly renew our

Program by addressing the everyday hurts and resentments that can lead us back to food.

11. Sought through prayer and meditation to improve our conscious contact with God, *as we understood Him*, praying only for knowledge of His will for us and the power to carry that out.

The Big Book teaches that, "As we go through the day we pause, when agitated or doubtful, and ask for the right thought or action. We constantly remind ourselves we are no longer running the show. We are then in much less danger of fear, anger, worry, self-pity... as when we were trying to arrange life to suit ourselves."[5]

12. Having had a spiritual awakening as the result of these steps, we tried to carry this message to compulsive overeaters, and to practice these principles in all our affairs.

We keep this Program by giving it away. When I share my experience, strength, and hope with another emotional eater, my Program is strengthened for my own self. I have to help others in order to hold onto my own recovery.

The Meetings

OA meetings can be used as a way to break through the isolation which is so typical of eating disorder sufferers. They are like a gathering of extended family where we can share our innermost selves and feel understood. We have to relate to one another in order to recover, replacing our self-contained world of food for the richness of human relationships. In the group, we can express the feelings that we short-circuited through food. We realize that we are not alone and that others share the weaknesses we have found so shameful and deplorable in ourselves. In *Fat is a Family Affair*, Judi Hollis discusses how "we have tried to get nurturance without being vulnerable. The only way to do that is with food."[6] The group teaches us to be vulnerable *without* food.

Telling our stories and having them witnessed by others helps us to grow and heal. When my grandmother died, the only place I was able to fully mourn was in my OA group. I felt my sorrow was too overwhelming for any one person to handle, and the wish to drown my grief in food was mounting. My pain was witnessed and contained by my friends in the OA group, and I felt "held" emotionally and deeply understood. My need for the food was eased.

The Tools

According to AA, "The alcoholic is absolutely unable to stop drinking on the basis of self-knowledge." Similarly for the food addict, self-knowledge brings us just so far and then it must be coupled with action. This is where the tools of the Program come in.

I am reminded of the documentary on chimpanzees by Jane Goodall, who points out that like humans, chimps are tool-using creatures. In her film we see a chimp sitting by an ant hill, watching very intently. He then picks up a stick that is lying beside him, inserts it into the ant hole, and gingerly pulls it out covered with ants. He then pops them into his mouth!

Despite the uncomfortable parallel with my own unwitting ant-eating episode in Spain, I was fascinated by this. Until the chimp picked up the stick and made it a tool, it was just a stick. It is in *grasping and using* the stick that it becomes a tool. It is in *grasping and using* the Program that it becomes a tool for recovery.

The Tools of the Program are:

The Food Plan: Rather than relying on the whim of the moment to dictate what I will eat, I pre-plan my food intake. This plan can be designed by a nutritionist or in conjunction with a therapist or sponsor.

Sponsorship: I work with one special person who is my guide. I check in daily with her to say what I will eat that day and "where I am at" physically, emotionally, and spiritually. Each day, I commit my food to my sponsor and am relieved of constantly obsessioning about when, where, or how much to eat.

The Slogans: These simple sayings have gotten me through the stresses of many days without turning to food. I have used them to center me, to calm me, and to remind me that whatever difficult situation is sending me to the food will pass, whether or not I eat over it. In the beginning, I felt silly reciting what seemed like nursery rhymes, but they worked, so I pushed through my embarrassment and reminded myself:

> *Easy Does It*
>
> *One Day at a Time*
>
> *I am powerless over other people, places, and things.*
>
> *Let Go and Let God*
>
> *First Things First*
>
> *Progress not Perfection is my Goal*
>
> *God grant me the serenity to accept the things I cannot change, the courage to change the things I can, and the wisdom to know the difference.*

The Telephone: I go for the call, not the compulsion, and in doing so, I break my isolation. I share with another "what's eating me" rather than "my eating it." Especially if I'm angry, I make the call to share my feelings. Actually, I coined a new motto for myself: "Better irate than I ate."

Writing: I go for the pen to discharge my feelings on paper rather than turning to food.

Readings: I bolster my connection with how others work the Program by reading what has inspired them.

Anonymity: I can speak my heart in a meeting and trust that my words will go no further.

Before I became involved in the Program, I referred to myself as an "alchemist in reverse." While the alchemist can turn anything into gold, I could turn gold into mud. I was able to see the negative of every situation, and this always drove me to food for relief. Through the Program I began to see the glass half full rather than half empty, and my emotional eating slowly subsided.

OA was the first leg of my journey in recovery. From the program I learned to substitute my consuming relationship with food for nurturing relationships with people, and I learned to work on my recovery on a day-by-day basis. Although eventually I traveled along a different path, my life has been immeasurably enriched by my connection with this Program.

CHAPTER 7

No More Diets, No More Deprivation

Freedom is when the bondage is understood.
—Krishnamurti

People who believe they are overweight, regardless of their size, are taught that the best way to control their eating is by dieting. Dieting becomes a lifelong project, perpetuating the daily obsession: "Was I good today?" "Did I cheat?" "How many calories did I consume?" "When will this diet make me thin?" "How much weight could I possibly have lost today?"

Whether it is the high-protein/low-carbohydrate diet or the high-carbohydrate/low-protein diet, the Rotation, Scarsdale, T Factor, or Carbohydrate Addicts Diet, we are bombarded with messages that promise: "Follow our plan and you will finally gain control of your food and your life." This seductive advertising implies that our anxieties and problems, many of which are out of our control, can be reduced to one neat and simple formula, "If I am thinner, I'll be happy. Therefore I should go on a diet."

Dieting is a camouflage—a detour. Instead of recognizing that our frantic need to diet is a coping mechanism for underlying emotional needs related to sex, anger, dependency, shame, and the fear of success, we simply adopt dieting as a way of life. But diets do not solve any of life's problems. They actually foster perpetual dissatisfaction with ourselves and trap us into a yo-yo cycle with our weight, the end result most often being weight *gain*, not weight loss. This is a fact that few diet plans admit.

Diets do not work! Rather, they teach us that we cannot trust ourselves and that we need an external authority to tell us what to eat. The implied message is that our hunger is dangerous, insatiable and must be controlled at all costs. Diets perpetuate our fear of food, invariably depriving us of the foods we most love. Since it is only human to feel that forbidden fruit is the sweetest, we wind up overeating, bingeing, or purging on the very foods the diets instruct us to avoid. If the latest trendy diet dictates that we can eat anything we want except bagels and cream cheese, guess what we will crave more than anything else!

Diets set up the following cycle which not only applies to binge eaters and bulimics, but also to those anorexics who have episodes of "break through" bingeing which punctuate their self-imposed starvation:

WE MAKE THE DECISION TO DIET

WE PUNISH OURSELVES BY
ADHERING TO A STRICTER DIET

WE ELIMINATE FOODS
CONSIDERED "ILLEGAL"

WE FEEL GUILT AND DISGUST
AT OUR WEAKNESS

WE FEEL DEPRIVED AND
CRAVE ILLEGAL FOODS

WE OVEREAT OR BINGE ON THOSE FOODS
IF BULIMIC, WE BINGE AND THEN PURGE

We were born perfectly self-regulating. We cried when we were hungry and ate until we were full. Hopefully, our parents responded to our signals and fed us on demand. As babies, we had not yet encountered the intense social and cultural pressure to be thin at all costs. We had not yet learned that stress can be temporarily assuaged by emotional eating. We simply ate when we were hungry.

This is the natural state we need to return to—feeding ourselves *on demand*. We need to relearn how to identify when we are hungry, how to permit ourselves to eat whatever we want without guilt, and how to stop eating when we are full. This is the philosophy of the **no diet/no deprivation approach**.

Hunger

Hunger is a complicated emotional, chemical, and physiological reaction which people experience in a variety of ways: rumblings in the stomach, feelings of light-headedness or fatigue, headaches, food cravings.

Hunger comes in varying intensities. Most of us go to extremes—either eating before we are actually hungry or letting ourselves get overly hungry. Paying attention to the nuances of your hunger by rating it can reacquaint you with your body's signals. The key to the non-dieting approach is to feed ourselves on demand at our body's *initial* signal of hunger. In the support groups I lead, we use the following rating system to help people interpret their degree of hunger:

0. **Empty**—feeling empty, famished, starving, dizzy, faint.

1. **Inner Nudge**—beginning to feel an inner nudge of hunger and the physical sensation of wanting to eat.

2. **Comfortable**—feeling comfortable, neither overly hungry nor overly full.

3. **Emotional**—feeling emotionally "antsy," anxious, in a tense state of wanting to eat.

4. **Out of Control**—bingeing, eating compulsively or purging, out of control, in the throes of addictive behavior.

Levels 0, 1, and 2 refer to the realm of physical hunger while levels 3 and 4 refer to the emotional realm. In my groups, I help people find alternatives to eating from levels 3 and 4. This work begins by trying to identify, "What are we *really* hungry for?" and "How can we best take care of this need?" The automatic reflex of reaching for food without being hungry will change only when these questions become an integral part of our self-discovery.

Each person has to discover his own unique way to feed himself on demand. Bruce was a young man who grew up in an alcoholic family where meals were erratic at best and often non-existent. The memories of hunger from his past continued to haunt him as an adult, and whenever he became physically hungry, he would panic and gorge all day long with no regard to how stuffed he felt.

In his struggle to overcome compulsive eating, Bruce committed himself to journal writing. Rather than reach automatically for food, he would grab for his pen whenever he felt discomfort and explore in his diary what was upsetting him. Over time, Bruce let go of the need to overeat throughout the day and was able to pause, let himself digest, and reach level 2—the comfort zone—before he ate again. Letting go of his need to feed himself all day was a courageous step for Bruce. And although he was still not able to allow himself to reach level 1, he was able to progress from nonstop bingeing to more of a recognition of his inner signals—a huge improvement.

Fullness

Just as there are stages of hunger, there are also stages of fullness of which we also need to become aware. Fullness levels range from:

0. **Empty**.
1. **Full enough**—Just full enough that the edge is off your hunger but you still want more to eat.
2. **Satisfied**—Feeling comfortable and satisfied both physically and emotionally with what you have eaten.
3. **Too full**—Have eaten too much and are quite full.
4. **Stuffed**.

Learning to stop eating when you are satisfied takes a lot of fine-tuning because feelings of fullness are never entirely predictable. Sometimes I am satisfied after eating lightly, and other times I am only satisfied when my belly is all filled up. Permitting ourselves emotional and physical satisfaction with *every* meal helps to avoid compulsive eating.

Many people know when they have had enough to eat but find it difficult to stop if there is still food on their plate. I call this "separation anxiety." I encourage patients to develop strategies that will help them "wave good-bye" to the food until the next time they are hungry. Other strategies to use when you are full but feel compelled to keep eating are:

• Take three more forkfuls "for the road" and really savor them. Then stop eating.

• Plan an after-meal activity that is a comforting transition away from the food—something to look forward to rather than a distasteful chore like cleaning up. Overeating is a great way to avoid the chores at hand. Leaving the table and reading a newspaper with your feet up on the couch is a perfect alternative.

• Create an after-the-meal ritual like brushing your teeth or saying a little thanksgiving prayer asking for the strength to stop eating.

Choosing Appropriate Foods

Not only do we need to tune into our levels of hunger and fullness, we also need to explore how to give ourselves permission to eat exactly what we are hungry for. No amount of cottage cheese will satisfy us if we are dying for chocolate chip ice cream. In fact, after eating the cottage cheese, we will probably go for the ice cream anyway.

The following is an exercise to help you determine the nuances of hunger:

1. Ask yourself if your stomach is hungry. Then wait for the answer. Are you thirsty? Often people mistake thirst for hunger. Try to tune in to this distinction.

2. Ask yourself if you want something hot or cold or room temperature.

3. Ask yourself if you want something creamy or crunchy.

4. Ask yourself if you want something sweet, salty, sour, spicy, or bland.

5. Now, ask yourself if your *mouth* is hungry. Does *it* want something hot or cold, creamy or crunchy, ...?[1]

6. From all the data and "feed-back" your body has given you, imagine the food that would best meet your hunger of the moment. Picture eating that food and "trying it on" in your imagination to see if it is, indeed, what you want to eat.

One patient of mine, delighted by this playful idea of asking for inner cues, decided to picture a disc jockey in her stomach taking requests! Whenever she became hungry she consulted her inner companion. It is actually possible to fine-tune our cues to such a degree that we can receive a very specific answer to our inner food requests. Another patient perfected this to the point that she knew exactly what she wanted on a particular evening: nothing else would do but mushroom pizza with peach wine!

You might ask, "What if my stomach is not hungry, but my mouth is?" This usually means you are struggling with an emotional hunger. When angry, for example, emotional eaters often like to bite and chew aggressively. When looking for comfort, emotional eaters will often seek out foods they can lick and suck.

Sometimes, despite all your best efforts, you may still have episodes of emotional eating, but this can offer you an opportunity to decipher what could have satisfied you instead. Were you angry, lonely, tired? How else might you have expressed or comforted yourself?

Abundance vs. Scarcity

When I was a teenager, baby-sitting for a family up the block with four young children, I remember gazing longingly into their kitchen cupboards and seeing a vast array of all kinds of wonderful food. I wondered what it would be like to live with a cupboard stocked for six people, and I pictured myself feeling the utmost contentment.

This is one of the key tenets of the no-diet approach— stock your cupboards and refrigerator with all the foods you love to eat. What if you love chocolate chip cookies more than life itself? Then go for it! Bring home ten boxes of cookies and replace a box each time you finish it. This can obviously be a very frightening concept for emotional eaters. "But I'll eat all ten boxes in one sitting!" they cry. While this may be true, and this is certainly not an approach that can be used by everybody, it is also true that human beings tend to relax and thrive when they live with abundance, and they tend to become anxious with scarcity.

Providing abundant food helps us let go of "the last supper mentality" in which we stuff down all the cookies right away because we are going on our next depriving diet tomorrow. When we are generous with ourselves, we also come to trust our self-parenting abilities. The principle at work here is that if we give ourselves the permission to choose from *all* foods whenever we are hungry, we will feel more free to say "no" to food when we are not.

The Body Nature Gave You

"Won't I gain weight if I eat everything I love, even if I learn to eat only when I'm hungry?" asks the emotional eater, fearfully.

The answer is complex. It is not simply compulsive eating but also repeated dieting that causes weight gain. Our body perceives any restriction of food as a threat to survival, and in response, lowers our thermostat to defend its fat reserves. This, in turn, slows down our metabolism, making it increasingly harder to lose weight. We all have an individual setpoint—the weight range that each of us is programmed to maintain. This setpoint is higher for some than it is for others, and that, it should be emphasized, is just fine. The best description of how this setpoint works and how repeated dieting thwarts our ability to lose weight is described in the book *Overcoming Fear of Fat*:

> I have witnessed a dramatic illustration of setpoint first hand with my cat who weighed seven pounds. She wandered away and was lost for about two months during which time she had lost half of her body weight. Following her rescue we noticed she no longer ate like a normal cat—taking a little food from its dish now and then. This cat ate voraciously. She ate everything in her dish immediately and continued to forage for more.
>
> My cat did not "lack will power." She was not depressed and she did not have emotional problems. She was hungry and her body, with a setpoint driven up by near-starvation, knew what it needed. Six months following her ordeal she weighed twelve pounds and was considered clinically obese. Her body became well-padded to deal with the next disaster. In her case, that would be getting lost in the woods again.
>
> In the fat woman's case, it could be the next diet.[2]

Feeding ourselves on demand will eventually bring us to our *natural* weight, the weight at which our bodies settle when we are not dieting, overeating, starving, purging or driven to compulsive exercise. Our natural weight is the weight we can maintain comfortably without rigid food restrictions or compulsive exercise.

Once upon a time in American history—the 1890's to be exact—a woman was considered beautiful if she looked like the actress, Lillian Russell. Voluptuous and buxom, Ms. Russell was considered the sexual icon of her day.

Times changed, and the era of the 1920's ushered in the flapper with a boyish, no curves body. Women actually bound their breasts to flatten them.

Then, in the 1930's, Mae West—curvy and ample—was the rage. No skinny flapper could have as convincingly declared, with a seductive roll of the hips, "Come up and see me sometime." In the 1950's, Marilyn Monroe was in vogue. Marilyn, the curvaceous sex symbol of her generation, wore a 12—a size that would be considered horrifyingly large by many women today.

The Twiggy era of the 1970's, like the 1920's, proclaimed, "skinny is beautiful." Twiggy at 5'7" weighed 92 pounds. In the 1980's, muscles for women made their debut. This style was followed by large breasts with no hips, then the worked-out and toned body and, currently, the waif look. And men are not exempt from the pressure to be lean and trim either. A New York gym, encouraging men to make themselves more masculine by working out their pectoral muscles, warns ominously, "No pecs? No sex!"

The moral of the story: We can *never* get it right, no matter how hard we try! If we looked like Twiggy when Mae West was in fashion, we felt unfeminine and inferior. If we looked like Mae West when Twiggy was in fashion, we felt the same way. Society is fickle. Body shape and size is a fad. Advertising and the media creates incessant self-doubt about our looks. We can manipulate our external image by dieting, starving, purging or exercising, but achieving the ideal "shape-of-the-day" does not guarantee inner peace.

Sometimes, learning to accept our body at its natural weight means accepting and even mourning the fact that we cannot achieve society's current (and shifting) ideal of perfection. Ultimately, declaring peace with emotional eating is an inside job. Living life to the fullest involves loving ourselves no matter what our size, and working from the inside out towards personal health and fulfillment.

Conclusion

Declaring peace with emotional eating includes the ability to maintain a comfortable weight that does not require undue strain. The focus, therefore, of the no-diet approach is to break the compulsive cycle of bingeing, starving, dieting, or purging. It is to respect and honor our body's signals of hunger and fullness.[3]

As an emotional eater myself, this was the path I eventually chose as the correct path for me. From my experience in Overeaters Anonymous, I had learned to calm down about my food and, over a period of time, I was able to regain control of my eating. The comforting, spiritual messages I had learned in the fellowship of OA became internalized, and I no longer felt the need to pre-plan my food or call my sponsor. I began to experiment with eating when hungry and stopping when full, and I learned I *could* trust myself. My appetite of the past—with its periodic rampages—no longer had a life of its own.

The no-diet/no-deprivation approach has now become my way of life. This is *my* story. But in my work with eating disorder patients, I have learned that there are many different paths to healing eating problems which I have come to respect as valid, depending on the needs of the individual person. Each of us must arrive at the approach or combination of approaches that works best on our journey to peace.

CHAPTER 8

Habits
Breaking the Chains that Bind

My very chains and I grew friends
So much a long communion tends
To make us what we are.
—Lord Byron
The Prisoner of Chillon

When I was a teenager, there were diet books that proclaimed that the best way to break the habit of compulsive eating was to put the fork down between bites and savor the food. By following this procedure, I was assured I could get by on less. When I tried this at a restaurant, the waitress came over six times to ask if I were done eating!

Other diet books recommended I eat without distraction—no reading, watching television, or driving the car; but my digestive juices never seemed happy unless I had a good murder mystery propped up in front of me during lunch. Still others went on to suggest I get into the habit of chewing my food twenty times before swallowing. Since I was already the slowest eater in the history of Western civilization, I was certain that if I ate any slower, I'd fall asleep with my head in the plate.

I was even encouraged to place a picture of my fattest self on the refrigerator door and dress in tight clothing to remind me of all the weight I needed to lose. But this always seemed like cruel and unusual punishment—not a way to feel better about myself or make positive changes in my life.

Eventually, though, I did discover helpful and supportive ways to change my eating habits, but these did not come from books. Rather, they came from an examination of my own thoughts and behaviors, and a willingness to trust my body's hungers. I came to recognize that I automatically reached for food whenever I was tired as a way of falsely energizing myself. In order to break this habit, I became willing to choose an afternoon nap as a healthy alternative to a banana nut muffin.

My other habitual pitfall included the conviction, "I can't believe I ate the whole thing, so I might as well eat even more." To break this thinking pattern, one which invariably led to my overeating out of discouragement, I replaced my thoughts with more encouraging statements. "So I overate. Let me stop now and put myself back on track. In 25 years, these extra chocolate cookies won't mean anything."

Habits enable us to structure our activities, organize our behavior, and even direct our thoughts. Thank goodness for the helpful ones which enable us to put the key in the car ignition and drive off without having to think about every step, or to brush our teeth automatically each night without having to be reminded. But we can also develop habits that are destructive to us—like smoking or spending money compulsively or emotional eating.

Certainly there are more complex and deeper issues contributing to disordered eating problems, but habits can become powerful influences which we must address and modify. Patterns of bingeing, starving, dieting, or purging easily become automatic. The clock strikes eleven, we turn on the television to hear the nightly news, and think, "It's time for some cereal and banana." Or, it's Saturday night, and we automatically go out to a restaurant and order a full course meal whether we are hungry for it or not. An anorexic might reject dinner after checking the fit of her jeans, or a bulimic might binge and purge every time she faces too much stress at work.

A habit is created in stages. Initially, we might make the decision to learn a specific behavior, or we might do something new that makes us feel better. If we repeat this activity many times, it can becomes automatic and our mind no longer has to think about it consciously. The bad news is that in the final stages, many harmful habits are deeply ingrained. The good news is that since habits are learned, we can "unlearn" them. We can replace hurtful habits with healthier behavior.

Identifying the Weakest Link

Clara was a school teacher who followed the same pattern each day. She would leave school feeling tired and hungry and walk home, stopping at the local candy store for the newspaper and a pint of ice cream along the way. Once home, she would consume the ice cream and fall asleep from the overload of sugar. When she awoke, Clara felt obliged to prepare dinner for herself and eat "like a normal person," even though she was not hungry. Since a chain is only as strong as its weakest link, we explored how best to break Clara's particular behavioral chain.

In the beginning we focused on breaking the connection between Clara's purchase of the daily newspaper and the ice cream. Since it appeared that these two things had become linked in her mind, we strategized that Clara should buy her paper during lunch hour and then walk home along a different route, thus avoiding the candy store and the ice cream. In her next session, Clara reported that she had done just what we had planned, but when she arrived home, she pulled out a box of cookies from the cupboard and devoured them in one sitting while she read her newspaper.

So much for scientific investigation! We went back to the drawing board and discovered that the *more* basic problem for Clara was feeling both fatigue and hunger when she left work. Realizing this, we planned another strategy. When Clara would come home, she would take a shower first thing, after which she would eat some yogurt and fruit and hop into bed with the newspaper. Often she would fall asleep, but when she awoke, she was refreshed and hungry for dinner. By taking the time to investigate the weakest link in her chain of behavior—her hunger and fatigue when she left work—and then trying out new strategies, Clara was able to break away from the daily ice cream habit which had kept her stuck and unhappy with herself.

Sandy presented a different situation. She was an actress, and each time she had an audition, she would eat large amounts of rice pudding and then repeatedly make herself throw up. Anxiety and emotional issues were, we discovered, at the core of her bulimia, but there was also an habitual component to her behavior that we needed to address.

Sandy's behavioral chain was as follows: She would buy the weekly show business newspaper and then come home to plan her auditions. Sometime during this planning process, anxiety would overcome her, and she would find herself rushing out to the store for massive amounts of rice pudding which she gorged and then purged. After she returned home from the audition, she would repeat this bulimic behavior with the rice pudding. It never mattered how well or how poorly she had performed—the habit remained the same.

Sandy's weakest link, we concluded, was choosing to go back to her apartment before and after the audition. Loneliness coupled with worry about her performance seemed to trigger the bulimia habit. We decided that Sandy should take her show business newspaper to the library instead of her apartment and plot her day from there. Following the audition, she was to return home with a take-out dinner and call me to report her day. The structure of these alternative behaviors proved extremely helpful.

Then an unexpected event further strengthened Sandy's ability to create better eating habits for herself. She had taken a trip to visit her family in the mid-West for Thanksgiving, and her mother had given her some old books from her childhood. Browsing through one of them, Sandy came across the following poem on a dog-eared page:

> "What is the matter with Mary Jane?
> She hasn't an ache and she hasn't a pain
> And it's lovely rice pudding for dinner again
> What is the matter with Mary Jane?

> What is the matter with Mary Jane?
> She's crying with all her might and main
> And she won't eat her dinner—rice pudding again.
> What is the matter with Mary Jane?"[1]

With surprise and delight, Sandy remembered how this had been a favorite poem her mother often read to her when she was a little girl. The memory of it and the fiesty spirit of the girl, Mary Jane, had been lost for over twenty years. Sandy began to see how she connected rice pudding with warm, happy memories of her mother and of her childhood, and she decided to read the poem aloud in front of the mirror before each audition. The comforting feeling of making this little-girl poem her own again replaced Sandy's frantic reach for the actual rice pudding.

Identifying Habitual Emotional Triggers

Certain emotional feeling states make people uncomfortable and can set off a habitual pattern of bingeing, purging, dieting, or starving. Identifying which states trigger your eating problems will help you become conscious of the times when you are most vulnerable. Rarely do people binge, purge, or starve for one reason alone, so you might find yourself in more than one category:

loneliness - using food to keep yourself company.

boredom - filling up empty time through bingeing or purging.

depression - seeking comfort or an "up" by abusing food.

preventive bingeing - overeating to protect yourself from being hungry at some future time.

anesthesia - using food, purging, or starving as a tranquilizer or to put yourself to sleep.

transitions - using food between activities to help you switch gears.

fatigue - using food to refuel yourself rather than resting.

lack of structure - using emotional eating to replace the missing structure of˙the work week, such as at night, on weekends, or on vacations.

separation/abandonment - using a connection with food to avoid feeling the pain of rejection or the loss of a loved one.

procrastination - using emotional eating to avoid or postpone the anxiety of some dreaded task.

fear of crying - overeating, starving or purging to avoid crying because it feels too painful or too indulgent; many bulimics throw up when they really need to cry.

avoidance of sexual intimacy - using food as a substitute for sex.

anger - biting, purging, or starving to discharge angry feelings.

retreat from people - obsessing about your relationship with food rather than risking intimacy with another person.

resentment - "swallowing" resentments and detouring them through emotional eating rather than confronting them directly.

happiness - believing that happiness is limited and needs to be gobbled up before it ends, or purged or starved out before it feels "too good to be true."

disappointment - using food to "make it up to yourself" for feeling deprived.

If you can learn alternative ways to handle the uncomfortable emotional feelings that are propelling you towards food, you will discover an amazing revelation: *Whatever inner feelings are prompting you to eat will pass whether or not you eat over them!*

Learning Self-Awareness and Self-Trust

Research has shown that it takes three weeks to discard an old habit and learn a new one.[2] This is an encouraging fact since so many of our harmful habits have become second nature and feel indelible after so many years of "practice." Learning self-awareness and self-trust are the first steps towards changing hurtful habits.

Diana had been laid off from her job and spent her days at home reading want ads and eating until she felt like bursting. "The other day I ate a whole chicken pot pie before I realized I can't stand them," she confessed to me in one therapy session.

"Well, why not try the following experiment," I suggested. "Try only eating food you really, really enjoy. And when you don't enjoy it anymore, just stop!"

No one had ever told Diana that she could eat for pleasure and she began experimenting with "enjoyment" as the guideline for creating new habits. Whenever she ate, she would periodically ask herself, "Am I still enjoying this?" Much to her surprise, she discovered that after the seventh bite of ice cream her mouth got too cold and she no longer enjoyed the dessert; the Italian food she was accustomed to overeating began feeling heavy in her stomach and did not satisfy her after a certain point.

With time, this habit of frequently checking in with herself became second nature for Diana, and she began to trust her ability to feed herself with care and concern. Automatically popping everything into her mouth was replaced by a respect for her own likes and dislikes. She even extended this habit of inner dialogue to other areas of her life as well, such as going out on dates and spending time with friends. "If I enjoy the experience, I go for it. If not, I stop!"

Other patients require different behavioral techniques. Mary was a young anorexic woman for whom food had become dangerous and frightening. Even the sight or smell of food made her afraid that she would become fat. But unlike many anorexics who feel some sense of triumph over their strict control of food, Mary was miserable. She was cold all the time, she could not find any clothes to fit her except in the children's clothing department, and she felt humiliated by comments about her thinness at work.

"Change is a slow process," I explained to her. "Is there anything at all about your eating habits that you would be willing to change?"

"Well, I guess I could begin by trying to make dinner each night," Mary replied with hesitation.

Knowing full well that dinner had always been Mary's least favorite meal and that her previous therapy had failed because her therapist had designed elaborate and structured eating plans for Mary, I did not want to overwhelm her. I knew it would be important for her to have an immediate sense of success. "Let's take it slower than that," I suggested, "by focusing on the easiest time of day for you and on the easiest change you are willing to make. Let's divide your anorexia problem into tiny, bite-size pieces and take it one bite at a time!"

Mary was willing to begin by eating fruit every morning. Although it may seem like a small, insignificant change, this was a definite first step towards altering her ingrained habit of avoiding food completely. What's more, Mary became an active partner with me in exploring what *she* was willing to do, and we inched our way along. Of course, there were deeper issues that we explored as well, but approaching Mary's behavior from the standpoint of habit modification provided her with concrete, successful steps to take.

Food and Mood Journal

To help people become aware of their habitual patterns of eating, I encourage my patients to keep a "food and mood" journal and become like Sherlock Holmes as they investigate what they have written. The following is a journal entry of one day in the life of Clara, the school teacher we met earlier.

TIME	FOOD EATEN	HUNGRY?	HOW DO YOU FEEL?
7:30 am	Coffee	No	tired, stuffed from last night
11:00 am	Coffee	Yes	anxious, overwhelmed by class
1:00 pm	Lunch: yogurt and fruit	Yes	still hungry, dreading afternoon
3:30 pm	ice cream	Yes	tired, wanting to relax
6:00 pm	Dinner spaghetti, meatballs, loaf of Italian bread, green beans	No	feel I should eat
10:00 pm	2 bagels with cream cheese, bowl of cereal	No	discouraged by how much I've eaten, depressed by my lack of willpower.

Question: What is the most prominent feature about Clara's pattern of eating?

Answer: Clara tries to be "good" during the day by following a strict low-calorie diet. Towards the end of the day, when she no longer has the structure and activity to distract her, hunger reasserts itself with a vengeance— ice cream, dinner, bagels, and cereal. Although Clara would never ask her car to run a whole day on an empty tank, she overrides and ignores her own hunger throughout the day. The next morning, filled to the brim, Clara starts the same habitual cycle all over again.

This particular pattern of eating behavior is so common that experts even have a name for it—"The Night Time Binge Eating Syndrome." I think a more apt name would be the "Vampire Syndrome." Deep inside of Clara and other problem eaters who make a practice of undereating during the day, lies a hungry, dormant vampire waiting to binge with great force once the sun goes down, seeking the next victim to consume, be it cake, a bag of potato chips, or the ice cream in the fridge. The habit of undereating or starving during the day is an inevitable set-up for out-of-control eating at night. By the same token, eating with satisfaction during the day is preventive medicine for compulsive eating at night.

For this reason, we needed to help Clara spread her eating evenly throughout the day. She began to include a full breakfast of cereal and banana or French toast which helped fortify her for the school day ahead. At midday, she would go out to lunch with her newspaper and have two slices of pizza or Chinese food. For a snack she would have her yogurt and fruit, and for dinner she would have some chicken and salad or fish and rice. Using the information from her food and mood journal, Clara found that *eating during the day helped her avoid bingeing at night*, and despite years of bingeing she no longer had the urge to do so.

Thought Patterns

Not only do negative behaviors become habitual, but the daily thought patterns and inner dialogues we carry on within ourselves also can become ingrained in hurtful ways. Below are several styles of thinking that emotional eaters "feed" themselves, creating self-destructive conclusions and feelings of hopelessness. Becoming aware of negative thoughts is an important step towards evicting them from our minds and being able to substitute more positive, supportive language.

Dichotomous Thinking is a fancy psychological term referring to the "all or nothing" mind-set with which emotional eaters often struggle. Either, "I'm 'good' on my diet or I'm 'bad.'" Either "I'm fat or I'm thin." Dichotomous thinking is also called black-or-white thinking because it leaves no room for shades of gray. "If I'm not perfect, I'm a failure!" Not only does this style of thinking permeate the emotional eater's reactions to food and her body, but it often extends to other areas of her life as well.

Instead of, "If I have ice cream I will never be able to stop myself from bingeing on it. I'll wind up totally out of control."

Substitute, *"I can have an ice cream and enjoy it. Only if I deprive myself will I start bingeing to make it up to myself and spin out of control."*

Superstitious Thinking involves linking together two ideas that are not related.

"If I eat this one cookie, I know it will make me fat."

"A cookie never made anybody fat. That's just my anxiety talking."

Over-generalization occurs when we apply to all situations what we conclude from just one or two experiences.

"Liz got the promotion I wanted at work because she's thinner than I am. I'll never get a promotion until I lose more weight!"

"I feel angry and hurt that Liz got that promotion. My usual tendency is to blame my weight for all my disappointments in life. What can I do now to support myself emotionally instead?"

Magnification occurs when we blow out of proportion the significance of a negative event in our lives and, at the same time, minimize our successes.

"I weigh more this summer than last. I can never go to the beach until I lose at least thirty pounds."

"I'm sorry I've had problems with my food this year and I need to look at what happened to me. But I won't let that get in the way of enjoying my summer to the fullest. I deserve to have fun regardless of my size."

Selective Abstraction means focusing on and drawing conclusions from an isolated detail of a situation even though there may be evidence to the contrary.

"My stomach got so bloated after lunch that I'm sure I've gained weight. How am I ever going to lose that fat?"

"Everyone's stomach gets larger after eating. The anorexic in me is so demanding. I know that when I'm through digesting my food, my stomach will go back to normal."

Personalization is thinking that all situations revolve around us. People with eating problems in particular tend to overestimate the importance of their appearance to others.

"Those guys were laughing when I walked by. They must have thought I'm fat and ugly."

"Who knows why those guys were laughing? My tendency to be mean and pick on myself makes me feel the whole world revolves around criticizing me!

Imperative Thinking refers to the perfectionist expectations we place on ourselves that dictate we are not allowed to deviate from a certain path. Our thoughts are peppered with "I should" or "I'll always" or "I'll never."

"I must exercise every day. If I don't work out today, I'll never do it again.

"Skipping a day or so of exercise never hurt anybody. I need to respect my fatigue and only work out when I'm feeling more rested."

Compassion Creates Healing Change

Our destructive habits and self-hating thoughts can keep us locked in a perpetual standstill. Often, to make ourselves feel better, we resort to our traditional methods of coping—overeating, purging, or starving.

Identifying and changing our negative habits is a process filled with fits and starts. When we can intervene in our own behalf with a generous serving of compassion, this process is made infinitely easier. Compassion, which means feeding ourselves supportive thoughts, paves the way for healing change.

CHAPTER 9

Psychotherapy
Getting Help with Healing

It takes two to speak the truth—
One to speak, and another to hear.
—Henry David Thoreau

Eating is a relationship—a relationship that can be either nurturing or abusive, supportive or neglectful, nourishing or punishing. Patterns of emotional eating often develop from the early patterns of loving in our family. If we have been hurt by the people we love, we hurt ourselves with food. Emotional eating becomes protection from pain.

In this way, eating disorders are really about our problems in human relationships. Detouring our need for love, connection, security, and intimacy through food is a way of bypassing our need for human sustenance.

People with eating disorders seek gratification through food rather than connection with people. Food, after all, is completely trustworthy and more compliant than any other relationship can be—it doesn't abandon, reject, or laugh at us, and it is always available when *we* say so. We get to say *when, how much*, and *where* without having to consult with anyone but ourselves!

When we binge, purge, or starve, we become totally self-sufficient and do not have to rely or depend on others. We try to become invulnerable because "a rock feels no pain. And an island never cries."[1] Only when we stop this emotional eating do we discover just how needy and vulnerable we really are, and that can be scary.

Healing an eating problem means learning to turn to people for nurturing rather than to our secret relationship with food. Psychotherapy is a powerful channel for this healing. In therapy we develop a partnership with another human being who is trained to help us unravel the inner reasons why we have made trusting food safer than trusting people.

Fear of Therapy

All problem eaters have fears when they enter therapy, especially when their relationship with food has felt like the glue that holds their life together. Joining a diet group or a fasting program does not create the same anxiety as going to a therapist, because in therapy we risk sharing our secret selves. "What will the therapist think of me?" "How can I reveal the shameful things I do with food?" "Will the therapist really understand?" "Can I really be helped?" "What if this is just another thing I fail at?" The fear of beginning therapy is exemplified in this letter written to me by a young bulimic woman:

> "I am a binge-vomiter and have been bingeing and throwing up for years but have never told anybody. I'm afraid to go for help because I'm really afraid to stop, and I'm afraid the therapist will try to force me to stop. I don't know what would become of me if I couldn't throw up. I feel desperate and alone. What should I do?"

And I responded:

"I want to support you for the courage it took to write your letter. I think this is your first step toward healing. Bulimia is not only a disease of bingeing and purging, but a vicious cycle involving shame, isolation, and withdrawal from life and people. Bulimia can be progressive, and you should allow yourself to get help as soon as possible.

"Because your problem did not begin overnight, you won't be able to resolve it overnight, nor would any therapist expect that of you. I think your worrying about what would become of you if you could not throw up means that the bulimia has 'helped' you rid yourself of some difficult, inner feelings. You worry that if you did not have that outlet, you would be swamped with those bad feelings. Actually, this is where a therapist can help.

"Therapy is a process that will enable you to gradually understand your feelings and find other ways to cope with them rather than with food. Therapy will also help you discover tools to undo the habits that have led you to binge and purge. You don't have to do this alone. You deserve to get help. People with bulimia usually are dealing with lots of feelings of anger and guilt that they need help 'digesting.' Of course you are afraid. Any change—even change for the better—can be threatening. A therapist is a special kind of friend who can appreciate and respect your fear, and yet gently work together with you to resolve this problem.

"Also, I want to take issue with your statement 'I am a binge-vomiter.' You are a human being with fears, hopes, and feelings. I wish you luck as you begin to unfold your unique human self."

Eating disorders serve to cover up fears. Secrecy, dependency, and abandonment issues underlie many eating problems to begin with, and the therapy relationship is bound to raise the same anxieties. It is only after some headway has been made in treatment and the behavior of bingeing, purging, or starving ebbs that a person comes to realize the degree this fear has played in his or her life.

Once these fears are acknowledged, the process of healing is set in motion. The courage to turn to a therapist to unravel one's problems is a first but crucial step in undoing the bond with food and replacing it with the bond of human nurturing.

Fear of Dependency

Many problem eaters are secretly afraid that underneath the sociable, independent person they present to the world is a little girl or little boy who wants desperately to be taken care of. This was the case with Kevin, a 35-year-old dentist who had come to see me because his binge eating was out of control. He was raised in an alcoholic home where both parents drank, and he had to become the parent to his younger sister. "I guess I became a dentist," he laughed ruefully, "because trying to get love in my house was like pulling teeth!"

Ever since he was a little boy, Kevin had assumed the position in life that he did not need anyone and could take complete care of himself. Instead of being able to turn to his family for soothing and comfort, he turned to food. When his weight began to soar, he realized something was wrong and came to therapy. Almost at once he found himself fighting against accepting my help and support. He was afraid that taking in even a little caring from another person would open the floodgates to a bottomless pit of neediness.

Kevin began to see how the push-and-pull between bingeing and dieting was a mirror image of the push-and-pull in his relationship with his wife, his children, and now with me. Before therapy he had steadfastly chosen "the secure comfort of food over the unpredictable comfort of other people."[2] But gradually he began to peek out from behind his armor of fat and food and turn to us for nurturing. His ability to finally let down his emotional guard with me became a turning point in freeing himself from his dependence on food.

Fear of Abandonment

Rose's mother had died when she was two, and as a reaction to this traumatic loss, Rose became anorexic as a teenager. She avoided attachments to people because, in her experience, the bond with her own mother had led to a devastating loss. She generalized that any need for an intimate connection would eventually cause her abandonment and grief. Even eating became a need that repelled her.

This steadfast independence was sorely threatened when she embarked on her therapy, and as our work became more important to Rose, she grew anxious that something would happen to take me away from her. Since Rose's mother had died in childbirth while having her younger sister, she was always looking for signs of my possible pregnancy and therefore probable death. During my summer vacation, Rose was sure the plane would crash. During the winter, she was sure I would get the flu and die.

All the fears of intimacy that had caused her to retreat from life into the carefully controlled world of calorie counting and self-starvation emerged again. However this time, when she relived with me the pain from her past, Rose was freed to grieve, to cry, to feel the depth of her hurt feelings again. Gradually, her trust in me grew and she began to let me and other people into her life, as well. With her increased ability to be nurtured by us, she began to nurture herself with food. Eventually, she ended her therapy with me knowing that our relationship lived on *within* her as a good, internal parent who would now guide and support her.

The Therapy Interview

Fear of the unknown often holds people back from seeking therapy. In order to demystify the process, I will describe below some of the questions I might ask in a consultation or first session with a patient, along with my reasons for asking these questions. Of course, no real interview is as structured as this, but these questions will give you the "flavor." [3]

After I consider the unique responses of each person to the questions, I begin to fashion a treatment plan which I share with the patient towards the end of our first session.

Your Present Situation

1. *Tell me what brings you here and how you hope I can help.*

In my opening question, I am trying to understand two things: Did you come to see me voluntarily or were you pressured by someone else? This gives me some indication of how willing or scared you are to begin therapy. I am also looking for your expectation of me. One man I interviewed told me he wanted my help to lose weight so he could win a bet at work! Treatment is most effective when the desire for change comes from within yourself and not from outside coercion.

2. *How did you feel about coming for this consultation?*

I want to learn something about your fears, hopes, shame, and anxiety. This will help me appreciate whatever inner resistance you had to overcome in order to seek therapy.

3. *Why are you coming for help now?*

I want to know if there are events in your life that have made you more in need of help at this time. Some people can make the connection themselves, others cannot pinpoint "why now?" although their problems can often be traced to a recent loss in their life. The death of a loved one, an illness, a move or a separation can cause people to become more vulnerable to developing an eating problem or can worsen an already existing struggle with food.

4. *What is a typical day like for you with food?*

I am looking for patterns: Do you eat very little during the day only to overcompensate at night? Do you nibble constantly throughout the day as if food were an intravenous tube?

Weight History

5. *What is your current weight? What do you want to weigh?*

Asking people what they want to weigh reveals how realistic a view they have of their bodies. When a very thin woman tells me she needs to lose twenty-five pounds, I know she is struggling with a body image problem that we will also need to address in therapy.

6. *What is the highest weight you have been as an adult? What was the lowest?*

I want to discover how you reached your lowest weight and whether it was stressful for you. This will help me get a realistic idea of your natural weight.

7. *What was your highest and lowest weight as a teenager?*

Many people's eating problems began during adolescence. I try to determine what might have been the trigger, such as a fear of one's developing sexuality or fears about leaving home.

8. *Did you have eating problems as a child?*

If you tell me your eating struggles began as a child, it indicates the problem may go deeper than the case of a widow, for example, who only developed a weight problem after her husband's death. A sudden weight gain or weight loss may indicate a traumatic event in the child's life such as sexual abuse.

9. *Were you ever teased about your weight? By whom?*

Getting weighed at school in front of the whole class or worrying about fitting into a gym suit are often painful memories for people. If a family member teased you about your weight, that will add to your pain and self-consciousness.

10. *Does your occupation require a certain weight?*

Patients who are dancers, actresses, flight attendants, aerobics teachers often come to therapy because their jobs are pressuring them to lose weight, and this is causing an unnatural obsession with food and eating.

Diet History

11. *Have you ever been on a diet?*

Dieting seems to be the norm in our society, especially for women. In my entire life, I have only met *four* women who never dieted!

12. *How did your dieting begin?*

I want to learn what role your parents played in your dieting. The mother of one patient forced her to diet at age ten, subjecting her to upsetting, weekly weigh-ins while her thinner sister was given free reign of the kitchen. This patient remained fat as a silent protest to her mother's intrusiveness.

13. *Do you have a way you prefer to diet? Do you fast, skip meals, take diet pills, or avoid certain foods?*

Generally, the more restrictive your method, the harder it tends to be for you to make peace with emotional eating; the more lenient the method, the easier it will be.

Binge History

14. *Have you ever binged? When did it start?*

Bingeing often occurs when two factors are present at the same time: You have suffered an emotional loss in your life and, simultaneously, you begin a weight loss diet.

15. *When are you most likely to binge?*

This will help identify the emotional state most likely to cause your eating problems. Is it loneliness, boredom, anger, depression, sexual tension?

16. *On what foods are you most likely to binge?*

Are there certain foods that provoke a binge such as cake, ice cream, bread? This alerts me to a possible addiction.

17. *Where are you most likely to binge—at home, at work, at school?*

Very often, the location or timing of the binge has a specific meaning for the person that, when understood, will help to break the cycle. One woman I worked with only binged in the bathroom stall at college. Another only threw up when she was going on a date.

18. *What is the longest you have gone without a binge? What helped?*

I want to know what support systems made it easier for you to avoid eating problems at that time.

19. *Do you binge around your menstrual period?*

If this is the case, I suggest that women increase their intake of complex carbohydrates and eliminate protein at the evening meal. This raises the body's endorphin level and reduces cravings.

Purging History

20. *Do you make yourself vomit? Since when? How often?*

21. *Do you take laxatives or diuretics? Since when? How often?*

22. *How often can you eat normally without purging?*

I want to understand whether you consider all foods dangerous or only certain foods must be purged. The wider the range of foods you consider forbidden, the more severe your eating problem may be.

23. *How often do you exercise? How compelled do you feel to exercise? Do you use it as a way of undoing a binge?*

I then ask about other related behavior:

24. *How often do you drink? Do you use drugs? Do you feel you ever had an alcohol or drug problem? What about spending too much? Shoplifting?*

Since so many eating disordered people are cross-addicted, this question rounds out the picture of possible substance abuse or other addictive behavior.

Family History

25. *Does anyone in your family suffer from alcoholism, drug abuse, eating problems, or depression?*

There are strong genetic tendencies among addicted families, one of which is depression. Eating disorders can be a symptom of depression and as such can be successfully helped through psychotherapy and possible anti-depressant medication.

26. *Have you ever been physically abused? Sexually molested?*

An alarming number of people with eating disorders have been abused as children. Food is the safest, most available drug for numbing painful feelings. If you have been abused, we need to address this gently but fully in therapy to help you heal your eating problem.

Rounding Out the Picture

27. *Have you ever been in therapy for an eating problem before? What was it like?*

If you were in therapy before, I want to learn what went right, what went wrong, and why you left. This can help me better understand your needs. The two most common complaints I hear are: "My therapist didn't talk to me enough. I didn't get enough feedback." And "I learned a lot about myself, but it didn't help my eating problem." My belief is that patients do not resolve their eating problems through insight alone. A therapist needs to be an active participant to help you weave together *both* your emotional issues with concrete strategies for changing your eating behavior.

28. *Is there anything that would be helpful for me to know that we have not discussed yet?*

I never fail to ask this question because some of the responses can be amazingly revealing. One patient "forgot" to mention that her son had died two years ago and her husband was beating her. Another patient "forgot" to mention that although she did not vomit outright, she would bring her food up and swallow it repeatedly.

Concluding the First Interview

In formulating a treatment plan for a new patient, two key elements usually emerge in the interview—one is behavioral and the other is emotional.

First, patients need a plan of action to begin giving some structure to their eating. To this end, I ask patients to keep a daily journal of what they eat, when they eat, whether they are hungry, and how they are feeling when they eat (or purge or starve). The second element that usually emerges is an emotional issue that has been camouflaged by the eating problem. I explain to new patients that therapy can be extremely helpful in unraveling and resolving these emotions.

Individual, group, and family therapy are the main avenues of treatment for an eating disorder. Let's first see how individual therapy can help.

Individual Therapy

Ellen, a divorced woman who had been bingeing and purging for 12 years, came for therapy when she was 36 years old. She was also depressed because her boyfriend, Joe, refused to make a more permanent commitment to her.

When we traced her episodes of bingeing and purging, Ellen became aware that they were often triggered by her feelings of intense rage and jealousy towards Joe. If they were at a party and he danced with another woman, she became furious. If he went to lunch with a female co-worker, she wanted to kill him. Unable to tolerate these hateful feelings, Ellen tore into food with a vengeance and then purged herself with violent spasms of vomiting. How could she wish such bad things on someone she supposedly loved?

In therapy, we discovered that rage and jealousy were issues for Ellen long before Joe came on the scene. She was the younger of two girls and was born with a deformed and shortened arm which required many operations and hospitalizations. When she expressed anger and grief to her parents about her handicap, they would reprimand her, "You should be grateful for all we're doing for you. We're spending money we don't even have to make you better." Their comments left Ellen feeling ashamed of herself, and she remembered beginning to secretly overeat at this time.

There was another feeling in her heart, though, which she could never reveal to anyone. It was a wish that *proved* what a terrible little girl she really was and that she deserved to be punished. She secretly hoped, "If only my sister Laura could have this ugly arm. Why did it have to be me? I wish *she* were the one."

This opened up a stage of intense grief for Ellen. She revealed how she never felt pretty as a little girl and that her arm had made her feel deformed and unlovable. She cried when she recalled how lonely she felt as a teenager at parties where she was afraid the boys would not ask her to dance. The long-sleeved blouses she wore, even in the summer when the other girls were wearing sleeveless dresses, barely disguised that her arm was shorter. Feeling like an outcast, she hated the other girls for their popularity.

Now it began to make sense why Ellen would fly into a rage when Joe paid attention to another woman. She feared that practically any woman was more attractive than she was, and that it was just a matter of time before Joe would choose else someone over her.

One session, Ellen brought with her the tiny brace she had worn on her arm when she was two years old. It had been wrapped in a handkerchief and kept in her drawer all these years. Looking at that cast together helped us appreciate just how little and tender and vulnerable Ellen had been when she went through this suffering. We began to understand why she had turned to food to comfort herself and how throwing up was her way of trying to rid herself of the inner, jealous feelings towards her sister and the other girls. It was also her way of trying to make herself feel clean and innocent and less guilty inside.

Through our relationship, Ellen was adopting my accepting attitude and beginning to view herself with the same compassion that I felt towards her. As she gradually became more accepting of her inner world, her need to hurt herself with food and vomiting subsided.

It was not until the following incident, however, that I saw how much Ellen had really used her therapy to grow emotionally. It marked one of the first times she was able to tolerate her own angry and jealous feelings without resorting to the self-punishment of bulimia.

A year into treatment, Ellen reported that her ex-husband, whom she had divorced five years before, was about to enter an alcoholism treatment program which she had not been able to get him to do all the time they were married. In one way, she hoped he would finally be successful and get sober since their children would benefit from having a more responsible, healthier Dad. But in another way, Ellen wanted him to fail. Why should his new wife reap the benefits when Ellen had suffered so much with him? Why should he get healthy now when he had never taken *her* advice in the past to get help? Voicing this in therapy helped her accept her vengeful feelings with a mixture of humor and rue, and she no longer felt like a monster worthy of her old punishment—bulimia—for harboring destructive feelings toward him.

With an increasing sense of self-esteem, Ellen also was able to discuss her hurt with her boyfriend, Joe, about his flirting with other women. Unable to appreciate her complaint, Joe criticized her for being "overly sensitive." Ellen, strong enough about herself for the first time and wanting more from a man than Joe was offering, decided to leave the relationship. It was one of the first times in her life she respected her intuition and honored her feelings about what she needed to do to feel good about herself.

Ellen's case illustrates the stages of psychotherapy for emotional eaters which we will discuss in more detail at the end of this chapter: **awareness** in which she learned to identify the emotions that had been responsible for her eating problems, **exploration** in which she came to understand the roots of these emotions and their connection with her past history, **grief** in which she experienced and mourned the original pain that she had stifled with her eating disorder, and **integration** in which she came to use these insights towards handling new experiences without resorting to the same hurtful eating behaviors of the past.

Group Therapy

Group therapy is another avenue of healing that can break through feelings of loneliness, isolation, and shame. A therapy group provides valuable feedback and a safe place to experiment with new ways of communicating and sharing. Members realize that they can be angry and still be liked. They can share their innermost shameful secrets, creating close mutual bonds with each other. This helps them "try on" new ways of reaching out to people for support instead of turning to the familiar "security" of emotional eating.

The group also becomes a "second-chance family" in which people have the opportunity to repeat and hopefully resolve the roles they held in their families of origin, but with a symbolic, supportive "cast of characters."

Sharing and Validating Feelings

The following is an excerpt from one of my groups which illustrates the support and validation that emerges in a group experience:

Christina: I finally had to admit to myself that I can't get into last winter's clothes, and I went to Macy's department store today to buy some skirts that will really fit me. I felt like such a failure to be up another size, but I also felt a commitment to get myself some nice clothes rather than waiting until I lose weight to feel entitled. It helped me remember what Frances said last week in group—that despite her weight, she still wanted to get the prettiest dress she could for her brother's wedding because if she didn't, she would feel disloyal to herself.

Frances: It's funny you remembered my saying that, because during the week I kept wondering why I had used the word "disloyal." Then I remembered that when I was growing up, my mother would come home with a new blouse or jacket for me which was always too small. They always just happened to fit my sister Gloria, and she would get to keep them.

I was horribly disappointed all the time. I felt my mother was being disloyal to me, that she really preferred shopping for Gloria but kept pretending the clothes were for me. I could never say anything to her, and she would do this again and again, and I would be disappointed over and over. I feel so angry at myself for not having the guts to tell her how much she hurt me. I was such a coward and that makes me mad at myself.

Judy: You're angry at *you* for not telling her off? What about *her*? It seems to me you have a right to be angry with her, not yourself. You had just as much right to get something new as your sister.

Frances: But I should have been able to say something. Maybe if I had told her how I felt, she would have realized how it hurt me.

Rachel: Frances, you forget you were just a kid. What were you supposed to do? You were probably too scared to tell her off. You act like you should have known how to be grown up and get her to change. If I ever dared complain about anything like that my mother would say, "You think *you* have it bad? When I was your age, I got nothing but hand-me-downs, so don't be so smart." I learned to keep my mouth shut.

Judy: And probably eat over it instead.

Frances: Well, maybe I am being too hard on myself. I think I once did actually say to her, "That's probably for Gloria," when she brought home a new blouse. But she looked so hurt that I felt bad for saying it. I guess I did try, but I didn't want to hurt her either.

Valerie: I can relate when I hear you say that you're angry at yourself for not speaking up. When I was nine, I had to wear chubby sizes and, with my luck, my Aunt Sylvia had a Chubbette store in Brooklyn that we had to go to! I was so humiliated. The store was dark, and the clothes were dark too. Aunt Sylvia and my mother would decide which outfits made me look thinner and which ones, as my mother would say, would hide "a multitude of sins." They always used that expression. But those "multitude of sins" they were talking about was my body! I felt like such a fat, ugly kid that I thought I had no right to speak up. I thought I was getting what I deserved because if I hadn't made myself fat in the first place, I wouldn't have to be there. How can you talk back when you feel it's all your fault?

Frances: You're right! I *did* feel that way. I never thought about it that way before. I thought Gloria deserved the new clothes more than me because she was thin. If I only would stick to a diet like my mother kept insisting, I could have new things too.

Judy: Well, it still makes me mad that you had to go through that...

Sandy: Please, could I say something? I never told anyone this before. (She starts to cry). When I was 12, I was very overweight and my grandmother bought me a girdle and a long-line bra to make me look thinner. The girdle dug into me so much it hurt. I knew I was the only 12-year-old in my class wearing one, and I felt like a freak. I can't believe I'm saying this. It hurts so much to remember.

Mary Anne: These are such painful feelings we are talking about. Even as little girls we felt ashamed of our bodies and our size, and the grownups in our life couldn't appreciate our pain about this. This is very sad.

When we were young, we didn't always have a way to express ourselves. We were dependent which made it hard to speak up. But here we are as adults with resources we never had as children. Now, we have to power to care for ourselves in more tender ways. Christina can now decide to go to Macy's and buy something really nice for herself. Frances can now say to herself, "Let me buy the prettiest dress I can for my brother's wedding regardless of what I weigh right now. I'm entitled to it and I want it." We can even turn to one another and get support, like saying, "I have to go clothes shopping, and I'm dreading it. Can we talk about it so I can make it easier on myself?"

Christina: That gives me an idea! I realize that what makes shopping so hard for me now is that I carry my mother's critical voice inside me, judging everything I try on. What if we did an exercise together where we pretend to go shopping with the good mother we all wished we had. Let's imagine what she would say to help us while we're shopping. That way we can create a new, encouraging voice to take with us instead!

Getting Needs Met

Group therapy also provides a unique opportunity to heal because the very reasons that people turn to food come alive in the group. Many compulsive eaters and bulimics struggle with the feeling that they are too needy, too greedy. This is a concern of so many people in the early stages of an eating support group that it seems to me that many of the women must have been born to the same family! They all tend to think, "I can only get love by taking care of others. I shouldn't be selfish. I want to be liked by everybody. I shouldn't take too much time for myself."[4]

Sandy: I've been very depressed since Dave and I broke up. I know I've been talking about him week in and week out, and you're probably all tired of me by now. Even my cousin Janice said last night, "All right, already. When are you going to get over him? He's not worth all this time and energy." I felt totally hurt and cut off by her, and so I started stuffing down donuts.

Rachel: You know, your problem is not just that you're depressed about breaking up with Dave. Your problem is that you turn to the wrong people for support. You remind me of a saying that my grandmother used to use, "Don't take your bucket to a dry well." You need to take your bucket to someone who's going to be able to understand and respond to you—not like your cousin.

Frances: I agree. You're so apologetic that you're burdening people even here in group, that you wind up choosing someone who tells you off. And then you overeat to console yourself!

Judy: (Changing the subject) Listen, I need to talk tonight before the group is over. Were you done talking?

Sandy: Yeah. I hear what you're all saying.

Judy: I had this major fight with my girlfriend last night, and I need to talk about it. Pam has been going through a rough time with her husband, and she had the flu, but she wasn't too sick to borrow my movie projector. When I told her I needed it back... (she trails off as she sees Valerie looking very thoughtful and sad). What's the matter, Val?

Valerie: Sorry, I wasn't paying attention. I was just thinking how bad I feel about what Sandy was saying about her cousin. I know that feeling myself of trying to get sympathy from someone who's critical. But go on.

Judy: (Faltering) I can't remember what I was just saying!

(All eyes turn on her in surprise).

Frances: You were talking about the fight with your friend and her borrowing your movie projector.

Judy: (Directing herself to me) Why can't I remember what I was saying?

Mary Anne: You "stopped remembering" right after Valerie said she was thinking about Sandy. Why do you think you forgot just then?

Judy: (Slowly) I guess I thought Valerie was criticizing me by implying I hadn't given Sandy a chance to finish talking.

Mary Anne: So...?

Judy: So I guess I thought she was saying I was a selfish person—that I was bad to interrupt her.

Valerie: I didn't mean that.

Mary Anne: Why don't you ask Sandy if she felt you were being selfish?

Judy: Did you?

Sandy: No. Actually I was done talking. Trust me. This group is the one place where I could tell you off if I thought you were interrupting me!

Mary Anne: But what if Sandy *was* angry and upset with you for interrupting her?

Judy: I guess I'd feel like I had done something really terrible—like I was being insensitive.

Rachel: You act like being insensitive is the same thing as committing murder! You could say to her, "I didn't realize I was interrupting. Please continue. I just wanted to make sure I get time for myself tonight, too."

Judy: (Starts laughing) You're not going to believe this, but what just happened here in the group was exactly the same problem I had last night with my friend Pam. She told me I was selfish for wanting my movie projector back when she was in the midst of all her problems. I felt maybe she was right—that I wasn't being understanding enough. The only difference is last night I ate over my guilt and tonight I'm talking it out instead!

Mary Anne: Let's look at what's going on here. Sandy feels guilty for burdening her cousin with her problems with Dave and eats over it. Judy feels guilty for wanting her movie projector back and eats over it. We seem to be grappling with a lot of inner feelings about not being entitled to our needs, that our needs are selfish. But look how food problems kick in when you feel you should shut up! So, let's talk some more about how it came to be that everyone here feels so selfish and guilty about claiming their needs and then winds up eating.

Family Therapy

Eating disorders do not develop out of the clear blue. They are born and develop within a family context, and for this reason, family therapy can be extremely helpful.

Families that have trouble setting boundaries, expressing their needs or anger, or allowing each member to live their own separate life will often produce a family member with an eating disorder. Sometimes, more than one family member will play a part in maintaining the status quo. An anorexic patient once told me that "family unity" was so strong a belief in her family that she was not allowed a new pair of shoes unless her other two sisters needed them as well! Her own unique needs and wishes were not respected by her family, and she translated their attitude into "if you are not going to listen to me or take care of me, then *I'm* not going to take care of me either." Her anorexia became a silent protest to their indifference.

An eating problem can also provide a way for families to avoid more threatening issues, such as the marital problems of the parents. The eating disorder becomes a safe battleground for the family when, in reality, the parents' conflicts with one another are the more basic problem. This was the case in the Collins family.

Ashley, age 11, preceded her parents into my office looking quite grown-up and self-contained. She looked like a miniature Shirley Temple doll, exquisitely dressed, very polite and almost intimidating in her adult presentation. In contrast, her parents, Renee and Steven, looked beaten down and tired as they followed her. Renee explained that Ashley had lost quite a bit of weight over the summer. Their pediatrician had expressed concern over the dramatic weight loss and suggested that the parents seek help.

In our first session, Renee and Steven pleaded with Ashley to tell me why she was having eating problems and Ashley, in full control, said she *liked* her stomach flat.

What's more, she wanted to weigh even less and not be forced to eat certain foods. I could see there was a role reversal in this family. Renee and Steven looked to their daughter for direction and guidance. When they begged her to tell them what they should do to help her, Ashley rose to the occasion and dictated to her mother that she needed to learn to cook *only* low calorie food.

At this point, I jumped in to block Ashley's tirade against her Mom. I turned to the parents and asked, "Why don't the two of you tell me what's been happening to make you both look so tired and worn out?"

Steven responded, "Ever since Craig was born two years ago, we haven't gotten a good night's sleep." Describing how their son's asthma and bronchial problems had kept them constantly on their toes, he added, "Ashley's had to fend for herself a lot more that she used to. My wife and I have really been tied up. It's also been a financial drain on us since I've opened my own art supply store." Steven looked at his daughter ruefully.

"But Ashley *loves* to be grownup," added Renee. "She's always been like that—so independent."

"Sometimes I think we push her too hard though. Her school marks, her gym team..." Steven added.

"That's ridiculous," countered Renee. "When I was Ashley's age, I was cooking and cleaning for my brother and sister. Who do you think shopped for food if not me?"

I glanced over at Ashley and was surprised to see her looking very much like a little girl. She seemed to enjoy having her parents talk about her. "Why was that?" I asked Renee in surprise. "How come so much of the responsibility fell on you?"

"Well, it was nothing really," she answered, uncomfortable that she had even brought it up.

Ashley piped up, "We wouldn't have any problems here if Mom wouldn't insist I put butter on my toast or eat red meat."

"Ashley," I said, "I know you are concerned about having to eat foods you don't want, but you jumped in just when your Mom was telling us what it was like for her at your age." I was aware that Ashley had tried to detour the conversation toward food in order to protect her mother. I wondered what she was protecting her from.

Renee continued. "My father was drinking heavily at that time and so was my older brother. Dad hit my mother a lot, and I tried to keep the younger ones out of the way." She paused. "There were other things, too."

And then I knew. Her indicating "other things too" led me to imagine another piece of the family puzzle. I invited Renee and Steven to come back for another session, this time without Ashley.

In our next session, Renee and Steven entered my office quite cheerfully. "Ashley's been eating more!" they exclaimed almost in unison. "Meal times at our house have not been so filled with problems for the past week."

Although I do not believe in magic cures, I sensed that Ashley might have felt more taken care of by her parents. Their coming to therapy on her account made her feel reassured and cared for. I recognized also that Renee's and Steven's cheerfulness served the same purpose as their daughter's interruption during the last session when Ashley, unaware of what she was doing, had tried to divert the family from confronting Renee's pain.

Renee and Steven continued to talk about Ashley's eating when I interrupted, "Last session, you talked about when you were Ashley's age."

Renee bowed her head and, after a few moments, said in a low voice, "When I was 12 years old my father and brother began touching me sexually. They made me do things to them I don't even want to talk about." She began to sob.

"I just found this out," Steven quickly added. "Renee only told me about this two months ago when we had to fly to her hometown in Virginia for a family wedding. I always suspected something was wrong because Renee always puts off having sex with me. She never seems to enjoy it, never seems to want it, and I could never get her to tell me why."

What emerged from Renee's story was that she had kept her shameful secret painfully wrapped up inside herself. She felt so damaged that she had not even dared to reveal herself to her husband. Tearfully, she continued, "When the pediatrician told me that the breast tissue Ashley was beginning to develop had disappeared after her weight loss, I remember thinking, 'Oh good. That gives her some reprieve. She'll grow up soon enough.' "

As Renee, Steven, and I continued working together, more of the pieces of the family puzzle came together, and we better understood the family context that had provided the fertile ground for Ashley's eating problems. Renee was able to reveal her fears about sex and began to realize how she had unconsciously transmitted this to Ashley. At the same time, Renee had a compelling need for Ashley to be perfect in her school work and in sports, as if she were requiring Ashley to compensate for her own self-doubts and feelings of inadequacy.

Spurred by his wife's courage, Steven also had a secret that he needed to reveal. As a younger man, before marrying Renee, he had had several homosexual relationships.

Although Renee had known about this, she did not know of the self-doubt that continued to haunt him. It now became clearer why Steven had tolerated Renee's asexuality in their marriage. His own problems with sexual identity made it safer for him to be in a relationship with a woman who was not very interested in sex. Ashley's coming of age also brought up anxiety for Steven because he wondered if he could be a masculine-enough role model for her.

This couple worked hard to undo the burdens of shame and guilt they both carried locked inside, and as a result, they began to recapture the vitality that had been drained from their marriage by the secrecy of their inner problems. This new openness also made them available to parent their daughter more actively. Once a month Ashley joined us for family sessions. In time, she became livelier and less robot-like, sometimes behaving like the little girl she still was, and at other times, like a healthy, somewhat obnoxious pre-teenager!

Ashley had turned to dieting and calorie counting as a way of feeling a sense of control over the unspoken anxiety in her family. Her weight loss was an attempt to slow down the clock and give herself some "time out." Although she knew nothing of her parents' past, this family—as do all families—communicated many key issues to each other nonverbally. Through the process of family therapy, Renee and Steven were able to claim and face their own pain without diverting it through their daughter. As a result, each family member began to bloom more in their own right.

The Stages of Psychotherapy

The stages of psychotherapy for emotional eaters often follow a certain course whether the person is in individual, group, or family therapy. I have identified four stages which most patients need to pass through in order to recover: awareness, exploration, grief, and integration.

Awareness

In the awareness stage an important change happens—you begin to observe yourself and your eating patterns. This seemingly small level of awareness can be a significant first step towards real and lasting change because, rather than taking your pain with eating for granted, you see how it has colored your whole life. You admit you are out of control, and an inner chafing for change begins.

Many people work hard to deny that food is making their lives painful and unmanageable. Perhaps this is your story too. Hopefully, at some point, you will come across a helpful book on eating disorders or see a friend change and grow through therapy. This begins to offer you hope that change is possible.

Exploration

In this stage, you start to realize how inner un-named feelings have caused you to reach for food as a way to soothe and comfort yourself. You begin to take a risk and tell your story. At this point you need to reach out to safe, supportive people who will acknowledge your pain and help you learn to trust again. As you become able to share yourself, your feelings will unfreeze, you will realize you are not alone, and the feeling of being "on the outside looking in" begins to diminish.

Grief

This grief stage is often the turning point in the recovery process because it hurts, and the temptation to return to emotional eating looms very large. In the grief stage, you are mourning for your inner child who felt hurt and betrayed and who learned to rely on the comfort of food more than relationships. Grieving is also the way of legitimizing your pain, by saying, "I am justified in feeling angry and hurt."

Jenny's father had died from a drug overdose when she was five, and she described her fat as "frozen grief." "When I was ten" she said, "I had an experience that was unbearable to me. My mother had just come out of a drug rehabilitation program. She and I found a baby robin on the sidewalk with a broken wing and we brought it inside to nurse it back to health. My mother put the bird on the stove and turned the heat on low to warm him up, but when I came home from school, the bird was lying dead on the stove. She had forgotten to turn the heat off. I felt destroyed, and no one could understand the depth of my reaction. People said "But, Jenny, it was just a bird."

When I came to the eating support group 30 years later and began telling my story and my struggles with overeating, those memories of the bird came back. It occurred to me that I had felt like this little bird—that despite all my mother's good intentions, she was unable to really care for anyone, herself included. These memories of the bird made me experience for the first time the shock and fear I had felt about my father's death. The little robin had seemed so tender and helpless. That bird was like my tender self that had to go underground with food because I could not trust anyone to take good care of me."

Integration

In this final stage, you learn to trust your own inner voice and intuition. You can identify and express your needs without shame and have found ways to fulfill yourself without retreating to your eating patterns of the past. You no longer feel driven to be perfect, but rather have compassion for yourself. This capacity for self-forgiveness helps you empathize and trust other people, as well. You learn to look at your foibles with humor rather than harsh judgment, and in your relationships you find a comfortable balance between dependence and independence.

The Therapy Relationship

To every patient's surprise, the relationship they develop with their therapist will often start to parallel the relationship they have with food. This connection with the therapist becomes a mirror to better understand their inner world of emotional eating, providing a rich avenue of exploration.

The eating styles of the anorexic, the compulsive eater, and the bulimic reflect the kind of relationship each develops with the people in their lives.

The Therapy Relationship and the Anorexic

The root of the anorexic disorder, in which the person prides herself on avoiding food and denying hunger, is directly related to the person's early family relationships.

Jody was a tiny sparrow-girl who had been anorexic since age 12. She told how her father held court at the dinner table each night, lecturing his children, lecturing his wife, raising his voice, and intimidating his family. Jody's stomach would close up with tension at these times, but her father forbade anyone to leave the table until they cleaned their plate. Usually, she forced herself to finish by choking down her food.

This was only one of many painful memories Jody had of her father's domination over the family. Now in her early 20's, she led an isolated life with few close friends and also greatly feared her boss at work. Although she appeared emaciated, Jody came to therapy not to be helped for anorexia, but for the deep loneliness and emptiness she felt inside.

Whenever I offered support and understanding to her in our session, Jody withdrew from me. It was as if my words made her wince. Then I realized that she experienced my words, like her father's, as being *forced* down her throat. She felt obligated to "swallow" my interpretations. How could I help her, though, if I couldn't communicate?

I began experimenting with silence, and I discovered that the less I talked, the more Jody slowly came alive. Because her experience had been that her body, mind, and soul were the possessions of her father, to receive an interpretation from me was to confirm her sense of inadequacy, as if I, too, were telling her what to think and feel. But when I became more passive, Jody took the reigns of the sessions rather than feeling "force fed" by me. As she came to control more of the therapy space we shared, Jody also began eating more. Finally, feeling more in control of both her eating and her relationships, she was slowly able to let go of her need to fend off food and other people.[5]

The Therapy Relationship and the Compulsive Eater

Compulsive eaters relate to their therapists in a variety of ways. Many feel they cannot "get enough" from the therapist. They demand, "Tell me what to do. Give me advice. Talk to me." Feeling deprived, they turn to the food and to the therapist to fill up the empty place inside. Some complain that their previous therapists did not talk enough, leaving them feeling cheated and hungry for more. Obviously, my role as therapist in this case is not to fill my patient up by chatting incessantly, but to try to tune in when she is feeling deprived and try to understand what is bringing about her feelings of emptiness at that moment.

Some patients work hard at guarding *against* this hungry inner self in order not to burden the therapist too much. I know I am sitting with this kind of "defensive" overeater when I start feeling bored. My own boredom alerts me that my patient is struggling to keep her distance from her own emotions and from me. She relates intellectually as if reciting an essay entitled, "My Emotional Problems," which is her way of protecting us both from what she believes is her unbearable, repulsive neediness.

This was the case of Janet, an obese 33-year-old gay woman who had been a compulsive eater since childhood. Shortly after she was born, her mother became ill, and she was sent to live with her grandmother. When Janet was two, her baby sister was born, and she was again sent to her grandmother's for several months. Then, when she was five, her mother began having outbursts of rage, pulling Janet's hair and hitting her with a wooden spoon.

Through her therapy and her relationship with me, Janet realized that she believed she was bad for needing and wanting too much. She was convinced that her voracious appetite for care and attention had driven her mother away. Overeating became an effective way to divert and disguise this need for sustenance from others.

In Janet's eyes, I quickly became Ms. Perfect Therapist. I could do no wrong. Janet would pull her chair up close to mine in my office and scrutinize my face attentively. As we got to know each other better, we learned that one meaning to her searching my face was to determine whether or not I was angry at her. Just as she had feared her mother's explosions, she now feared mine. And even though we kept working on Janet's overeating and bingeing, she found no relief.

Then, after my summer vacation, which came at a difficult time for Janet because her grandmother was dying, I began to have the impression she wanted to bite me, both to extract more emotional milk/nourishment and to express her anger that I was not there when she needed me. Evidently my vacation had brought up feelings of abandonment and old bruises about being left alone, but Janet was too afraid to reveal her anger towards me. So she continued biting into food instead of "biting" me.

Following a particularly needy session in which she was upset about her grandmother's illness, she asked, "When will you be taking your next vacation? I think you should take one soon."

"What makes you ask about my vacation at this point?" I inquired.

"You look tired and probably need some more time away from your patients," she said.

I said, "You feel that your neediness drains me, and you are sucking me dry..."

She interrupted, "I feel I want so much from you that you should go away and restore yourself."

"It's as if you feel I have a finite amount to give you and that you may use it up," I continued. "You are scared of wanting too much from me—that I will get angry with you and pull away from you."

Although she continued to be terrified of her voracious feelings, a gradual shift occurred in our work together after this session. Instead of constantly asking, "Is our time over yet?" which meant "I am afraid I have been a bad girl and taken too much from you," she began to ask, "Do we have some more time left?" I understood her rephrasing the question to mean, "I am able to admit that I have hungry needs and I want more from you. Maybe I'm not so bad to admit that I want more."

As Janet was gradually able to take in my soothing presence and to know that I accepted her even when she was angry, she was able to interrupt her own binge with new-found coping methods. She began turning more to me and to her friends rather than gorging on food.

The Therapy Relationship and the Bulimic

The bingeing and purging pattern of the bulimic also parallels her style of relating to people. She will let herself get close to someone only to eventually reject and dismiss them, banishing the relationship from her system just as she does the food. A most astonishing example of this occurred in my initial evaluation with Amanda, who informed me over the phone that she had been bingeing and vomiting for the past thirteen years.

From the first moment we met, Amanda hated me. She said I looked like her last therapist, Ms. G., who had abandoned her practice to join a cult religion. Ms. G. had written a letter to Amanda saying her job on the commune was to scrub toilets, and she felt uplifted in a way she never had as a therapist! Amanda had decided on first viewing that I could not be trusted—just like her bulimic self had decided many years before that food could not be trusted. Reassurance that I would not abandon her abruptly nor leave her to scrub toilets (I barely had time to tend my own!) would have fallen on deaf ears.

In this initial consultation, Amanda told me that because of my resemblance to Ms. G., she could not trust me nor did she want to work with me. I was actually her third therapist, and I remarked to Amanda that she seemed as bulimic in her relationships with people as with her food—always trying to get rid of us. "But I do not expect you to trust me," I said. Some of her other therapists had tried to convince her they were indeed trustworthy, while I recognized that Amanda's "not trusting" position was exactly where she needed to be in this beginning relationship of ours.

So we began on this rocky road, and as Amanda's therapy unfolded, she confided what life had been like for her when she was growing up. She had adored her handsome father and always turned to him for comfort when she was little even though he drank too much. But when she was six, as she lay cuddled in his arms, he began to fondle her sexually, stroking and rubbing her body all over.

Amanda's world shattered to pieces. Her father's betrayal had destroyed forever her innocence and trust. He had turned on her and had become poison, just like later in life, food—the comforting nurturer—had become poison as well. This mistrust of her father not only spilled over to food but to all her relationships as well. Now, her suspiciousness was reflected in her relationship with me, her therapist.

For this reason, our relationship became *the* avenue to discover and explore Amanda's inner world. Every time she wanted to leave therapy and "spit me out," we worked on tracing back what had triggered this new episode of mistrust with me. For the first time, she was able to express her wariness without worrying that I would be angry or retaliate. This translated into her ability to trust her food as well, and hold it down. Understanding these parallels between her early life, her food, and her apprehensions also gave Amanda a sense of relief that she was not just "crazy" but that her behavior had rhyme and reason.

Just as the disappointments we experienced with the people we love became the original reason we turned to emotional eating, so must human relationships be the path toward our cure. The courage to turn to a therapist to unravel one's problems is a crucial first step in undoing the bond with food and replacing it with human nurturing. As Shakespeare writes,

"Give sorrow words; the grief that does not speak
Whispers the oe'r fraught heart, and bids it break."[6]

Emotional eating has frozen our feelings and pains. Relationships can help us thaw.

CHAPTER 10

Medication, Mood, and Mallomars

Even the most winged spirit
cannot escape physical necessity.
—Kahil Gibran

"If I take medication, aren't I just turning to a pill as a crutch the way I've always turned to food? Aren't I just substituting one dependency for another?" This is the question patients most often ask when I suggest that medication might be helpful for their eating disorder.

My answer is that medication does not perform miracles, but in certain cases, it can be a powerful tool to help a person make peace with emotional eating. Many of my patients who have been on medication have said to me: "I used to be so depressed. All I wanted to do was binge and sleep. I felt a heavy curtain between me and the rest of the world. Now, that curtain has lifted and I feel hopeful for the first time in ages. I feel more like the me I used to know!"

Throughout this book I have emphasized the significant role that emotions play in creating an eating disorder. It is important to add, however, that not all eating disorders stem from emotional issues. Our complex internal biochemistry also controls our eating patterns and our perceptions of hunger. Sometimes, unless our inner chemistry is regulated, we may not have the resources to face the underlying emotional issues surrounding our eating problems.

Over the past twenty-five years, scientists have made great strides in understanding how the brain works. Their research points to the enormous role that hormones, neurotransmitters, and enzymes play in affecting our behavior.[1]

The pathways in the brain that regulate our eating behavior are made up of chains of nerve cells. Messages are passed from one cell to another by chemicals called neurotransmitters. If there is a chemical imbalance in the brain because of an abnormal level of neurotransmitters, these pathways can go awry and lead to eating disorders and/or depression. Medications such as anti-depressants can be used as a way of re-regulating the amount of chemicals in these brain pathways. They "remind" the body of the correct route in order to become balanced again. Rather than being a crutch, therefore, medications gently nudge one's inner chemistry back to a more normal state.

Researchers have also discovered that certain foods influence the chemicals in our brain which directly affect mental energy, mood, behavior and performance. Foods rich in carbohydrates, for example, serve as natural tranquilizers. They can trigger the release of neurotransmitters which, in turn, elevate our mood and make us feel better. So when we binge on mallomars or bagels we may actually be trying to medicate ourselves for anxiety or depression without even knowing it. Mallomars do lift the spirits—but only temporarily.

Medications for Eating Disorder Behavior

Medication can be beneficial for eating disorder patients in several different ways. In some cases, they target and alleviate the eating disorder behavior directly. In others, they relieve the symptoms of depression, anxiety, obsessive compulsive disorders, or premenstrual syndrome that often accompany and even give rise to eating disorder behavior. In still other cases, medication provides a combination of effects by relieving some of the eating disorder behavior as well as the underlying symptoms of depression, anxiety, or obsessive compulsive disorders.

Bulimia

The biochemistry of bulimia is the most researched of the eating disorders. Bulimia is:

(1) Recurrent episodes of binge eating (rapid consumption of a large amount of food in a short period of time).

(2) A feeling of lack of control over eating behavior during the eating binges.

(3) The binges are usually followed by purging by self-induced vomiting or overuse of laxatives, diuretics, or enemas. Non-purging bulimia involves strict dieting or fasting or vigorous exercise in order to prevent weight gain.

(4) A minimum average of at least two binge eating episodes a week for three months.

(5) One's self-evaluation is unduly influenced by body shape and weight.

(6) Bulimia nervosa can be divided into the purging type or non-purging type (fasting or excess exercise).[2]

Of the three major eating disorders, bulimia has proven to be the most responsive to treatment with medication. Both depressed and non-depressed bulimics seem to improve with anti-depressant medication which can significantly reduce the urge to binge and purge.

Binge Eating Disorder

Binge eating disorder is what most people think of as compulsive overeating. However, it was not considered a specific medical diagnosis until 1994, when it appeared for the first time in the psychiatric literature. Because of this lack of recognition as a disorder, there has not been as much research on the treatment of binge eating with medication.

Binge eating disorder refers to "recurrent episodes of binge eating in the absence of the regular use of inappropriate compensatory behaviors characteristic of Bulimia Nervosa." In other words, unlike bulimia where the person "gets rid" of the food they have eaten, the person with this disorder "keeps it."[3]

In the past, most notably during the 1960's and 70's, people flocked to their doctors for appetite suppressants such as diet pills and pep pills—commonly referred to as "speed"—to help them lose weight. Not only did these people regain their weight once they stopped taking these pills, but these medications had a highly addictive potential. Diet pills also caused sleeplessness, anxiety, and even psychosis. Although they are no longer considered an acceptable treatment for binge eating, the *New York Times* recently reported an upsurge in the use of diet pills among ten-, eleven-, and twelve-year-olds.

Some evidence indicates that compulsive overeaters who binge out of control because of a specific "attack" (experienced as an immediate need to stuff down food) can be helped by the same medications used to treat bulimia. However, if someone is constantly overeating throughout the day without that specific "attack" of craving, medication may not be as effective.

Anorexia Nervosa

By anorexia nervosa we mean:

(1) A person refuses to maintain normal body weight and instead continues to maintain a weight less than 85 percent of the normal expected weight for that person.

(2) Intense and inordinate fear of gaining weight or becoming fat, even though underweight.

(3) Disturbance in the way in which one's body weight, size, or shape is experienced, undue influence of body weight or shape on self-evaluation, or denial of the seriousness of the current low body weight.

(4) In females, absence of at least three consecutive menstrual cycles when otherwise expected to occur.

(5) Anorexia can be a restrictive type (self-starvation) or alternate with bingeing and purging.[4]

Restoring an anorexic's weight to a more normal range is crucial because malnutrition itself can lead to the symptoms of depression, confusion and obsessive preoccupation with food so often seen in these patients. With adequate nutrition, some or much of the anorexic's depression may abate. Once the malnutrition is overcome, it is possible to evaluate more accurately which of the anorexic's symptoms were related to physical starvation and which are emotional and need to be dealt with in psychotherapy.

For the last three decades, researchers have tried to use appetite stimulants to increase the food intake of anorexics. These efforts have largely failed because anorexics are, in fact, hungry. Their problem is not a lack of hunger, but their resistance to these hunger feelings. The last thing an anorexic needs is to have more hunger feelings generated.

There is no clear indication that medication can be helpful in directly reversing the anorexic's starving behavior, but, in certain cases, researchers have hypothesized that the anorexic may respond to the same medications as the obsessive compulsive because both are constantly preoccupied with perfectionism and driven by obsessive thoughts.

Medications for Related Symptoms

As mentioned above, eating disorder patients experience a high incidence of depression, anxiety, panic disorder, obsessive compulsive behavior, and premenstrual syndrome. Medication can often relieve these symptoms which will, in turn, diminish the eating behavior.

Depression

Research now shows that almost three quarters of all patients with anorexia and bulimia suffer from a depressive disorder.[5,6] Clinicians report that a significant number of compulsive eaters also suffer from depression although there are no direct scientific studies to prove this.

Biologically based depression, which is related to abnormal chemical functioning, is different from the normal emotion of depression that many of us feel from time to time. It is sometimes difficult to distinguish what is biologically based without professional help. Indeed, at times, an emotional depression can actually trigger internal chemical changes.

Types of Depression

There are several types of depression:

A **major depression** refers to an acute episode of depression lasting more than two weeks with five of the following symptoms:

(1) depressed mood

(2) a lack of interest or pleasure in life

(3) a significant weight loss or weight gain not related to dieting

(4) an increase or decrease of appetite every day

(5) insomnia or oversleeping every day

(6) psychomotor agitation or retardation every day (feeling "hyper" or "dragged out")

(7) fatigue or loss of energy every day

(8) feelings of worthlessness, or excessive or inappropriate guilt

(9) diminished ability to think, concentrate, or make decisions

(10) recurrent thoughts of death, suicidal thoughts, or suicidal behavior[7]

Dysthymia or **depressive neurosis** refers to a chronic state of depression that has lasted for at least two years. Even the person's achievements and successes do not alleviate the depression, except temporarily.

Bipolar depression is a disorder in which the person's mood swings between lows and highs, ranging from deep depression to inappropriate elation (formerly called manic-depressive illness).

Atypical depression tends to be chronic and more common in bulimics. Symptoms include increased appetite, weight gain, bingeing, oversleeping, heaviness in the arms or legs, and sensitivity to rejection, particularly romantic rejection. (It is called atypical depression because it is the opposite of typical depression which usually involves loss of appetite, weight loss, and insomnia.)

Seasonal Affective Disorder (SAD) is another form of biological depression often connected with eating disorders. It resembles atypical depression, but only occurs during autumn and winter months and abates with the increase of sunlight in spring and summer. Seasonal Affective Disorder responds to light therapy and MAO Inhibitor medications.

Types of Medications for Depression

Many different kinds of chemical abnormalities underlie the various depressions, so there are many types of medications used to treat them. Sometimes a trial period is needed until the most effective medication for each person is found.

Tricyclics (such as Elavil or Tofranil) were some of the first drugs to be used to treat depression and have continued to be used for 35 years. They have been the traditional medication for the treatment of this disorder and have been the standard against which newer treatments have been measured.

MAO Inhibitors (such as Nardil or Parnate) were introduced about the same time as the tricyclics and appear to be particularly effective in the treatment of atypical depression. These medications require that a patient comply with special dietary restrictions, such as avoiding red wine or aged cheese, which can cause dangerously high blood pressure. Doctors may not want to use these medications with those binge eaters who have trouble following dietary instructions.

Lithium is used to treat manic depressive illness and to enhance the effect of other anti-depressants. Blood levels of this drug need to be carefully monitored to achieve the correct therapeutic effectiveness. Seventy to 80 percent of manic depressive patients respond favorably to lithium.[8]

Prozac first appeared on the market in 1987, and since that time, has received a tremendous amount of press coverage. Prozac, like many of the other anti-depressants, has proven to be highly effective and has few side effects. It is relatively easy to find the right dose for each patient, and unlike many other anti-depressants, it usually does not cause weight gain. In fact, patients taking this drug frequently report weight loss and increased feelings of control over their eating. Prozac is particularly effective for the treatment of bulimia because it tends not only to lessen the urge to binge and purge, but also to relieve the depressed mood of the bulimic person. More than 15 million people throughout the world have had Prozac prescribed for them.

Concern has been raised in the media that Prozac contributes to suicidal or homicidal feelings in certain patients, but this has been largely dismissed. A small group of patients report feelings of jitteriness which can make them feel as if they are worse. Prozac, therefore, as with all medications, needs to be carefully monitored by a physician.

Panic and Anxiety

Patients with eating problems often suffer from panic disorders and anxiety. Panic attacks refer to a sudden explosion of physical symptoms such as heart pounding, shortness of breath, or trembling, accompanied by a sudden fear of impending death or insanity. These attacks feel very intense—coming on suddenly, peaking to a crescendo, and then disappearing in about ten minutes. They often occur for no obvious reason. A panic *attack* occurs sporadically, while a panic *disorder* refers to a specific amount of attacks per week occurring on a regular basis.

Many eating disorder patients also experience anxieties such as social phobia (fear of being in social situations), simple phobia (fear of a specific object like snakes or spiders), agoraphobia (fear of going outside), or obsessive-compulsive disorder. Some experience anxieties which are related to persistent dieting, such as anxiety about losing control of their eating or anxiety about being too fat. Anorexics have a significant percentage of anxiety disorders and studies of bulimic patients report that over 50 percent have at least one anxiety problem.[9] Patients who suffer from panic disorders and anxiety can be helped with an anti-depressant medication such as Prozac, tricyclics, or MAO Inhibitors, as well as anti-anxiety medications such as Xanax or Ativan.

Premenstrual Syndrome

Premenstrual syndrome (PMS) refers to a wide range of symptoms that women suffer during the week prior to their monthly period. For many women, premenstrual syndrome often worsens their eating problems, although these symptoms usually abate dramatically a day or two after the onset of the period.

The symptoms of PMS include irritability, tearfulness, depression, anxiety, difficulty concentrating, increased alcohol or drug use, and food cravings. They run the gamut from quite mild to severe enough to impair daily functioning. In a recent study at the Premenstrual Syndromes Program at New York's Mount Sinai Hospital, 85 percent of the women described symptoms of depression and 56 percent reported cravings for carbohydrates.[10]

Before considering medication, there are certain measures you can take to reduce the stressful symptoms associated with PMS. Altering your diet during your PMS week by eliminating or reducing caffeine, nicotine, alcohol, sugar, and salt, decreasing your dairy intake, and replacing animal fats (such as butter) with vegetable oils (safflower, corn) can all be helpful. Many women also report improvement in PMS symptoms and bingeing by eating small meals every three to four hours.

In addition, increasing the amount of carbohydrates in the diet will also provide relief. Carbohydrates increase the level of serotonin, one of the endorphins in the brain which contributes to our feeling calm, and PMS has been associated with lowered levels of this chemical. It has been found that to get the most effective use of the carbohydrates, they are best eaten without protein, which can dilute their effect.[11]

Another way of improving PMS without medication is regular exercise three times a week, lasting at least 20 minutes. Aerobics have been shown to reduce symptoms because exercise increases the endorphin level in the brain and therefore improves mood.

If these changes in diet and exercise do not sufficiently alleviate the PMS symptoms, then medication should be considered. Anti-depressant medications like tricyclics, MAO Inhibitors, and Prozac have all been reported to be effective. Before embarking on drug therapy for PMS, however, one should first rule out underlying medical, gynecological, and psychological conditions with a physician.

Considering Medication

How do you decide if *you* can be helped by medication? The first step is a consultation with a therapist. In my practice, I always try to determine the severity of a patient's state of mind and mood to see whether we should first give psychotherapy a chance or proceed with a medication evaluation right from the beginning.

If the situation is not urgent, my recommendation is to begin a trial run of therapy. I would blend behavioral work, which focuses on habits to help you get back control of your eating, together with psychotherapy, to address the emotional issues underlying your eating problems. If there is no change in your eating behaviors after this initial therapy (about three months), then I suggest a consultation for medication.

However, if the situation is urgent at the outset—your depression, anxiety, or panic are out of control, or if you are struggling with suicidal impulses, alcoholism or drug abuse—then a medication evaluation is required. This type of evaluation would also be required if you have anorexia with life-threatening weight loss, or medical complications due to bulimia. Sometimes a hospitalization is necessary to help someone stabilize this type of crisis.

If your therapist is a non-medical professional, such as a social worker or psychologist, and an evaluation for medication is indicated, you will be referred to a psychiatrist who is a medical doctor, licensed to prescribe medication. Your therapist and psychiatrist will then work hand-in-hand to help you.

During the evaluation, the psychiatrist will review the background of your eating problem as well as other emotional, physical, and behavioral symptoms you may be experiencing. The doctor will also review your past psychiatric, medical, and family history, because addictions, mood disorders, and anxiety disorders are often hereditary.

It is especially helpful to work with a psychiatrist who has expertise in the treatment of eating and mood disorders. For instance, the commonly prescribed dosage of Prozac for depression is 20 milligrams a day. However, it is now known that many patients with bulimia do not respond to this dose, but may respond to a higher one of 60 milligrams a day. A doctor with expertise in eating disorders will know that anti-depressants will not be as effective for patients with a sluggish thyroid, and thyroid medication is sometimes needed as a booster. Thyroid medication may even be prescribed for those patients who have normal thyroid function to boost the effect of the anti-depressant medication.

Just as with psychotherapy, medication requires a certain length of treatment, the usual course for depression being six months. A trial of less than six months may not be as helpful nor will the benefits be sustained for as long. If, after a six month period, the patient's eating disorder and mood swings are stabilized, medications can be tapered off. For psychiatric disorders other than depression, such as anxiety or obsessive compulsive disorders, patients should be placed on medication for a similar trial period.

Many patients are able to sustain the benefits after their first trial, but may occasionally relapse because the re-regulation of their inner chemistry does not persist. Medication then needs to be continued for another course of treatment. "Patients who do need to continue taking anti-depressants do so because their disease continues, not because they have become dependent on anti-depressant medication. A depressed patient who continues to need medication is dependent on it only in the same way that a person with high blood pressure is dependent on medication: he must control the symptoms of a continuing underlying illness."[12]

With all my eating disorder patients, I recommend a current medical evaluation by an internist or family physician and routine lab tests. The physical examination will look for medical conditions, such as thyroid or endocrine problems, anemia, hepatitis, mononucleosis, an ulcer, tumor, or other health concerns that could be affecting mood or eating behavior. A medical condition, such as described above, does not necessarily preclude taking psychiatric medications.

When Medications are Not Indicated

Medication is not the answer if you are merely looking for a diet aid for quick weight loss. Nor is it the answer if you have poor eating habits, have a medical condition that resembles a weight problem, such as hypothyroidism, or are actively involved with drugs or alcohol. Although active involvement with drugs usually requires treatment in a detoxification or rehabilitation facility first, most of the medications we have discussed are not habit forming or addictive, with the exception of certain anti-anxiety medications. If you *are* in recovery from alcohol or drug abuse, they may be taken safely under medical supervision.

Other patients who may not benefit from medication are those for whom the eating disorder has provided a "glue" for their very shaky sense of self. Some of these patients may get considerably worse if their eating symptoms improve too abruptly. In this case, medication would not be recommended.[13]

Medication—Worth a Try

Patients sometimes worry that their true feelings will be covered up by medications or that they will feel like "zombies" while taking them. This is not the case. Unlike street drugs, which create an artificial high or a lulling sedation, the medications we have discussed here help you *restore* your natural mood and balance.

Since some of these medications are relatively new, the jury is still out on their long-term effects. However, the evidence is reassuring. We do know, for example, that medications such as Elavil, Nardil, and Tofranil, have been around for a long time with no substantiated long-term ill effects. Prozac has had no long-term ill effects after many years of use in Europe, and lithium can be managed safely through routine blood tests.

Depression, on the other hand, usually gets worse over the long-term if left untreated. Not only does it cause severe misery for the depressed person and their family, but chronic depression causes a breakdown in the immune system that can lead to other illnesses. Trying to "tough it out" without medication may sound admirable, but, in many cases, will not provide relief. A biological illness does not improve through willpower.

If your therapist and doctor agree that you could be helped by medication, I believe it is worth a try. I also believe that medications alone are not as effective as medication coupled with psychotherapy, where you can tackle *both* the emotional and the biological components of your eating problem. There are many patients for whom I do not recommend medication at all, but increasingly, I have witnessed how medicines can better equip some people to more clearly address their emotional problems in psychotherapy.

Ongoing research in the field of eating disorders continues to shed light on the complexity of these syndromes and their biological underpinnings. Leaving no stone unturned to help yourself with your eating problems, such as a trial run of medication, can be a truly compassionate act on your own behalf.

CHAPTER 11

How to Plan
Your Own Path

The good life is a process, not a state of being.
It is a direction, not a destination.
—Carl Rogers

In one scene of Henry Jaglom's motion picture, *Eating*, a group of women are at a party to celebrate a friend's birthday when out comes the cake. Everyone sings, "Happy Birthday," the candles are blown out, and the cake is cut. The first slice is put on a plate and then passed from one woman to the next until it circles the room and comes to rest uneaten in a corner.

As the cake went by, I wondered what the women were saying to themselves:

- "I can't eat this—it's too fattening!"
- "I'm on a diet, and this will really blow it."
- "One bite won't be too much. But if I eat more than that, I can just get rid of it later."
- "I don't deserve to be eating this. I'm too fat anyway!"
- "I'm not eating if *she's* not!"

And on their way home, I wondered if they:

- furtively stopped at the bakery, to stock up on an assortment of goodies to make up to themselves for the cake they did not eat.
- went home, stood over the kitchen sink gorging on frozen pie from the freezer.
- went home, starved from how little they ate all day, and fell asleep, believing that a flat stomach is worth it all.
- went home, binged on cottage cheese and diet soda and made themselves throw up.

In the movie, the scene ends with two women who each keep and eat a piece of cake. One is the mother of the birthday girl, who is in her early seventies and who cannot understand what all the fuss is about. The other is a young woman who secretly takes her slice to a back staircase where she sits forlorn on a step and glumly downs the cake. She is later caught vomiting in the bathroom. (Sadly, the actress who played this part was, in reality, bulimic herself and died shortly after the making of this movie.)

Many people, like these women, are struggling with food as a way of life. They are either chronically depriving themselves of food or sneaking it on "back stairways." However, there is a wide range of satisfying alternatives to this depriving behavior, and this chapter will outline some of them so you will be better able to plan your own path to peace.

What's Best For *You?*

As we have seen from the stories throughout this book and in the scene from *Eating*, there are many different kinds of problems with food. In the same way, there are many different paths which lead to healing. People often fail to resolve their eating problems because they try to fit themselves into an approach that is not congruent with their needs. They do not take into account that they are unique, and that what works for another person might not work for them.

The first step in designing *your own plan* is to decide whether to start with an addiction or a no-dieting/no-deprivation approach. Then you need to explore your habits, both behavioral and thought patterns, and the emotional issues that trigger your food problem. Next you need to determine whether you want to try psychotherapy and/or medication. One of the best ways to make this determination is in consultation with an eating disorder therapist. Finally, you will need to discover for yourself what gives your life meaning beyond the food. This last ingredient will sustain your recovery in the long run.

It can be confusing to decide which approach will be most supportive for you. Actually, some people find that concentrating on changing their habits is all that is needed. Others need medication. Still others develop a blended approach combining the different elements that they feel are most relevant to their progress at that time.

As you read this chapter, try to see what resonates most for *you*. Keep in mind that as you change and grow, your needs may also change. Later, down the road, you may want to choose a different "a la carte" selection.

No-Diet vs. Addiction Approach

Particular confusion arises in deciding whether to follow the **no-diet** approach, with a reliance on one's ability to identify and satisfy one's hunger, or the **addiction** approach, with its external structure and twelve step support. Clear differences exist between the two. Let's compare and contrast what experts from each side would say:

The addiction approach says:

"Food addiction is a chronic, progressive and ultimately fatal disease. We are powerless over certain kinds of food."[1]

The no-diet approach says we do have power over food:

"The first step in breaking free... is to eat when you are hungry. Nothing has to be forbidden if you remain aware."[2]

Addiction therapists believe:

"It doesn't matter if you stay away from the binge food for months or years, the food will still trigger a binge."[3]

No-diet therapists believe:

"It has been my experience and that of my patients that a woman can, indeed, after much work and soul-searching, free herself completely and forever of an eating problem."[4]

Addiction experts say:

"Food is a drug. Every addict has to learn one day that the relationship is harmful."[5]

No-diet experts say:

"Each time you feed yourself when your stomach is hungry, you are nourishing yourself..." The cure is "to feed yourself on demand."[6]

In other words, the **Addictions Model** tells us that eating disorders are a life-long illness that cannot be *cured*, but only *arrested* one day at a time. Therapists holding this view believe that for some people, eating certain foods is a form of substance abuse, like drinking alcohol is to an alcoholic. They believe that eating disorders are a physical, emotional and spiritual disease, and they recommend the structure of a program such as Overeaters Anonymous, where there is support from others with similar problems. An OA type program would encourage you to choose a sponsor to help design a daily eating plan to eliminate dangerous binge foods.

On the other hand, the **No-Diet/No-Deprivation Approach** believes that eating disorders are indeed curable, and that eventually people can learn to eat normally by paying careful attention to their own inner cues of hunger and fullness. Therapists of this approach explain that structured food plans do not work because they deprive us of some of the foods we love, and set us up for an inevitable binge on those very foods.

How do we know whom to believe? Whose advice shall we follow? How do we finally choose what is best for us? Experts from each side believe *they* are right. So, who is?

The truth is they *both* are, but they both have left out the key variable in this controversy which is *YOU,* with your unique mosaic of strengths and vulnerabilities, needs and desires, heredity and beliefs.

Each person's eating struggle is as unique as a fingerprint. Every emotional eater is not created the same. What works for me may not work for you; and, as you saw from my story, what worked for me 20 years ago is very different from what works for me today.

The ultimate goal of either approach is to help you move increasingly from **reactive** eating, which is vulnerable to external stress, toward **responsive** eating, which is attuned either to your own personal food plan or to your inner physical hunger. Emotional eating is reactive eating. Responsive eating would be one of the following:

1) preplanning your meals with a structured food plan.

2) preplanning your meals with a structured food plan and then learning, in time, to eat when hungry and to stop when full.

3) learning to eat when you are hungry and to stop when full.

The Importance of a Compatible Approach

The experiences of Helen and Laura illustrate how two different eating disorder patients may be treated in the wrong way for the wrong reasons.

Helen was a compulsive eater who suffered from chronic depression. A few months before coming to therapy, her brother died of a drug overdose and, a month after that, her mother was killed by a motorcycle. Overwhelmed by deep feelings of grief, Helen began bingeing out of control.

When she came for help, her therapist, who adhered to the no-diet/no-deprivation approach, advised her not to restrict her foods, but rather to "legalize" the foods she loved. She was told to "tune-in to her inner self" and use her hunger awareness as a guideline to determine when she should eat and when she was full. Helen, whose life was in chaos at the time, was unable to "tune-in to her inner self," and her therapist's permissive advice frightened her. Her eating binges escalated, and she finally left therapy convinced she was a failure.

Laura had a different experience. She had never had problems with food before her baby was born, but after Kimberly's birth she became bulimic. Terrified she would never lose the weight she had gained during pregnancy, she began dieting stringently, which then led to out-of-control bingeing and purging.

Laura's therapist, who adhered to the addictions approach, told her that she had a disease, was powerless over food, and could not rely on her inner self to dictate when she was hungry. She recommended that Laura join OA where she would be taught the technique of planning ahead of time what she would eat, discuss her food plan with a sponsor, and learn how to arrest her addiction one day at a time by using the spiritual help of the program.

Laura was alarmed at her therapist's drastic view of her eating problem and was upset that her therapist implied that she would never be able to control herself. Discouraged that she could not meet the degree of commitment recommended by the therapist, Laura left therapy.

What went wrong that neither Helen or Laura could respond to their therapist's advice? Each women felt like a failure in trying to mold herself to an approach that was inappropriate to her real needs. Both were left with the feeling that something was wrong with them, when, in fact, they were struggling with a mismatched therapeutic approach.

When Helen came to therapy with me, she was desperate for some structure to contain her anxiety, grief and chaos. She could not concentrate on hunger, fullness, and the "legalizing" of all foods that the no-diet model recommends. So we encouraged Helen to become immersed in OA which helped her to structure her food. The Program also became a second-chance family for Helen at a time when she sorely needed it.

In Laura's case, dieting during the day backfired at night. For lunch she ate only a yogurt and coffee, and for dinner she ate a salad. After her husband went to bed, she raided the kitchen, bingeing on cookies and ice cream, and then, filled with disgust, she would make herself throw up. In her therapy, I helped Laura become more aware of her daily eating habits in order to break the pattern of undereating during the day and bingeing at night. In time, she resumed eating when she was hungry and was able to let go of her diet-binge-purge-diet pattern and return to a normal relationship with food.

Other people are helped by a *blended* approach. Rita was already in Overeaters Anonymous when she came to see me, but after one year of working together, she was able to internalize the ability to eat when hungry and no longer needed to rely on an externally designed food plan. She developed a compatible relationship with food she never had enjoyed before.

John designed another version of the blended approach. He recognized that eating sugar made him feel depressed for days and also set him up to crave more and more sweets, so he joined OA to help him become sugar-free. Every day he committed to his OA sponsor that he would not eat sugar. John also looked to the support of his "OA family" for an emotional and spiritual connection. Unlike Helen, who relied on a daily food plan to dictate what and when she would eat, John *was*, for the most part, able to rely on his own inner hunger to indicate what to eat, and he ate from a wide variety of different foods—excluding sugar.

My Basic Strategy

There are no specific rules for helping someone develop the best strategy for healing. I often use a combination of intuition and experience. In general, though, and with certain exceptions that I will discuss below, I start my patients with the most basic approach: I teach them about the no-diet/no-deprivation model, and I combine that approach with an emphasis on restructuring behavioral habits and thought patterns. Often, as in the case of Laura, a dramatic improvement takes place when a person learns the tools and techniques of tuning in and responding to physical hunger.

If this strategy is not helpful enough, I begin to explore the meaning of the eating disorder in the person's life and how it may help them deal with anxiety or depression. I encourage them to explore issues about the fear of success, and I especially look for unresolved issues of grief. I also consider whether medication could be helpful.

Finally, if someone is still actively in the throes of bingeing, purging, or starving, in spite of the work we have tried, I introduce the idea that the eating disorder may be an addiction—a physical, emotional and spiritual problem—that requires a daily commitment to OA and the structuring of a daily food plan.

This strategy of starting with basics (the no/diet approach and habit/behavioral work) and, if needed, moving to the more complex interventions (psychotherapy, medication, addiction model) is the general progression I follow with most people. However, there are certain exceptions which lead me to alter my usual plan:

• if a person's eating or weight is jeopardizing her health or life or if there is an alcohol or drug problem that is out of control, I will recommend hospitalization.

• if a person is deeply depressed and/or suicidal or the eating disorder has become life threatening, I will recommend hospitalization.

• if a person is struggling with bingeing, undereating, or purging and is also depressed, with sleep disturbances or difficulty functioning at home or on the job, I will begin immediately with an exploration of emotional issues and a possible medication evaluation.

• if a person is out of control with eating and seems too compulsive or panicked or anxious (as in the case of Helen) to absorb and utilize the education and information I have to impart, I will begin with the addiction approach and a recommendation to attend OA meetings.

• if a person is obese and/or has suffered from disordered eating for most of his or her life, I will begin with the addictions approach.

Sometimes in the beginning of therapy with certain patients, we cannot hit upon a clear-cut path. In these cases, I try to develop a composite picture of the person's health issues, the quality of their relationships, the kind of support system they have, their work history, their early childhood history, possible trauma, and their sexual relationships. The more deprived or impoverished the picture—if their problem is of long standing duration and/or affecting their health—the more likely I am to recommend a trial run of Overeaters Anonymous at the outset. The more enriched and organized the personality of the person and the more recent the onset of the eating problem, the more I am likely to recommend a trial run of the no-dieting approach. Together, we "try on for size" these different orientations until my patient begins to experience relief and comfort with the food.

As I have stressed before in this chapter, each person's eating struggle is as unique as a fingerprint; therefore, every solution to resolving the struggle is valid. The key ingredient is to identify the approach which helps *you* feel most at peace with *your* food and *your* body.

Planning *Your* Strategy

The following questionnaire will help you determine which is the best path for you. Circle the number of "yes" answers for each category and then count them. Make a bar graph of your "yes" answers using the blank graph below. If, for example, you have eight "yes" answers under the no-diet approach, then make a bar from number 1 up to number 8. Continue with the other categories.

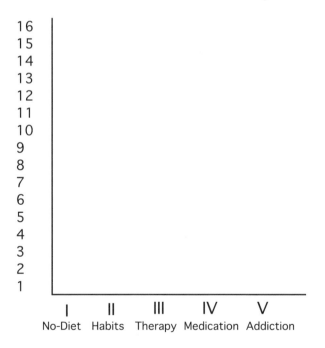

My own recovery from emotional eating took me from the addictions approach to the no-diet approach. As a therapist, however, I generally *begin* my work with patients using the no-diet approach and move in the order of deepening complexity—habits, therapy, medication, addiction—as needed. For this reason, the questions listed appear in that order.

Questionnaire

I. The No-Diet/No-Deprivation Approach

1. Do you generally know when you are hungry?

2. Are you comfortable letting yourself get hungry between meals?

3. Has there ever been a period of time in your adult life when you considered your eating normal?

4. Do you think you can eliminate "distracted eating" (in the car, following an upsetting conversation) so your inner hunger and fullness signals are clear?

5. Have you been able to stop eating when you are full without feeling unduly deprived or anxious?

6. Would you consider trying to legalize all foods— even your binge foods—if that meant you could finally learn to eat in moderation?

7. Are you ready to risk not going on another diet?

8. Do you have a support system of friends, family, therapy or a group to turn to for emotional support when you are under stress?

9. Can you risk stocking your cupboards with an abundance of the foods you love and replenish your supply each time it dwindles?

10. Can you permit yourself the flexibility of not eating at traditional mealtimes if you are not really hungry?

11. During your adult life, have you been able to maintain a normal weight for any extended period of time?

12. Are most of your close friends and family normal eaters?

13. During your adult life, have you been comfortable with your body size and shape for any extended period of time?

14. Do you have the capacity to enjoy food without undue guilt?

15. Are there things in your life that give you pleasure beyond food?

16. Are you tired of depriving yourself of the foods you enjoy? Would you like to reintroduce them into your life?

II. Habits

1. Are there certain times of the day you are more likely to binge, purge, or starve?

2. Do you undereat during the day only to binge at night? (Or undereat during the week only to binge on the weekend?)

3. Have you dieted repeatedly only to find yourself bingeing and regaining your weight?

4. Are there certain people, places, or situations that trigger an automatic response of emotional eating—bingeing, purging, or starving?

5. Are there certain inner emotional stresses that trigger you to overeat, purge, or starve, such as boredom, anxiety, loneliness?

6. Do you accuse yourself of being a failure on any given day if you have trouble with emotional eating?

7. Are you obsessed with weighing yourself?

8. Do negative thoughts about your eating habits or your body dominate your thinking?

9. Do you restrict your activities (going to the beach, dating, looking for a new job) because of how you feel about your body?

10. Do you feel your eating habits or patterns are abnormal or embarrassing?

11. Do you clean your plate whether or not you are hungry?

12. Does a party or holiday or weekend automatically mean you will binge or purge or starve?

13. Do you avoid social situations because you will be forced to eat?

14. Do you judge and criticize yourself after a bout of emotional eating and feel you need help becoming more compassionate to yourself?

15. Are you willing to increase your exercise habits? (This question does not apply to anorexics or exercise bulimics.)

16. Are you willing to try alternate behaviors to emotional eating and self-monitor yourself through journal writing?

III. Psychotherapy

1. Does depression, anger, anxiety, loneliness, or sexual tension trigger emotional eating problems?

2. Do you find yourself sabotaging yourself as you begin to succeed in resolving your emotional eating?

3. Do you come from an alcoholic, physically abusive, or addictive home?

4. Have you been sexually abused, incested, or raped?

5. Does emotional eating interfere with your work, family life, relationships, or sexuality?

6. Do feelings of shame or guilt dominate your thoughts?

7. Are you aware of feelings of not being entitled to happiness or feeling that you deserve punishment?

8. Have you recently experienced the death of a loved one, a rejection, illness, or difficult separation?

9. Are you aware of feelings of unresolved grief?

10. Do you suffer from compulsions? Panic attacks? Phobias?

11. Do you have difficulty knowing or expressing your inner needs and/or feelings?

12. Do you feel unfulfilled in love, work, or family relationships?

13. Do you have a family history of being criticized or made fun of for your weight or eating problems?

14. Do you have power struggles with your parents or your mate about your eating?

15. Do you believe that people would not love you if they really knew you?

16. Do you feel fat even though people tell you that you are normal weight or too skinny?

IV. Medication

1. Are you a compulsive overeater who experiences your need to binge and stuff down food as an "attack" that comes on all at once?

2. If you are bulimic, do you persist in bingeing and purging despite having addressed your eating problem in therapy for at least three months?

3. Do you suffer from depression?

4. Do you struggle with feelings of worthlessness or guilt?

5. Does your mood swing between highs and lows?

6. Do you often feel overly sensitive to rejection?

7. Do you become more depressed during the autumn and winter months only to feel better in spring?

8. Do you suffer from regular panic attacks in which you become short of breath, tremble, and fear you are about to die or go crazy?

9. Do you have any phobias—such as fear of leaving the house or fear of social situations—that interfere with your life?

10. Do you have any compulsions or rituals that interfere with your everyday life?

11. Do you suffer from monthly pre-menstrual syndrome and tend to have more eating problems at that time?

12. Do you have a family history of depression, anxiety, or mood disorders?

13. Do you have a family history of addictions—drug abuse, alcoholism, gambling, eating disorders?

14. Have you had a major loss in your life—the death of someone you love, a romantic rejection, the loss of a job—from which you have had difficulty recovering?

15. Do you have feelings of wanting to hurt or kill yourself?

16. Do you have problems with insomnia, early morning awakening or sleeping too much?

V. Addictions

1. Are there certain binge foods over which you feel powerless—once you eat them you just crave more and more?

2. Has emotional eating been a long-term struggle for you since childhood or adolescence?

3. Do you have any other addiction besides food? Alcohol? Drug abuse? Excess spending? Smoking?

4. Is there anyone in your family with a history of obesity, compulsive eating, alcohol, drug abuse, or gambling?

5. Are feelings of isolation, shame, or loneliness a large factor in your eating problems?

6. Do you consider yourself addicted to food, exercise, throwing up, laxatives or diuretics?

7. Do you ever lie to people about what you eat or what you weigh?

8. Does your eating, purging, or starving interfere with your work, your relationships, your family life, or your sexuality?

9. Do you find yourself consuming ever-increasing amounts of food?

10. Do you have withdrawal symptoms if you cannot get your binge foods—crying spells, insomnia, irritability, difficulty concentrating, depression, anger, fatigue, or headaches?

11. Do you have any health problems due to weight? Vomiting? Laxative abuse? Excess exercise?

12. Do you seek out the euphoric feeling associated with fasting or exercising?

13. Is eating, dieting, exercise, purging, starving, or worrying about your weight the main focus of your life?

14. Have you ever taken diet pills for an extended period of time?

15. Do you feel your eating is out of control?

16. Do you have frequent weight fluctuations greater than ten pounds?

Tally all of your "yes" responses for each category, and complete your own bar graph on page 204.

Sample Bar Graphs

Let's look at some sample bar graphs of the people we have met in this chapter. Helen suffered from depression and compulsive overeating all her life, and the death of her mother and brother deepened this depression, causing her eating to spiral even more out of control.

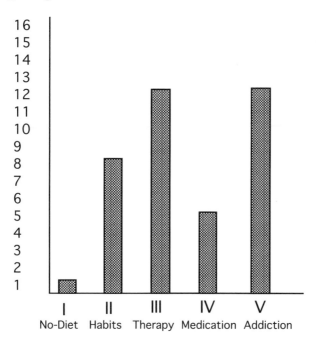

From her bar graph above, it was clear to us that Helen was an addictive eater who could be helped by the support of OA. Her emotional issues were also considerable, so for her, we blended a combination of psychotherapy, medication and habit/behavioral work. This turned out to be the most suitable choice because the fellowship of OA, the comfort of therapy, and the assistance of medication helped Helen find relief from her depression and her eating disorder.

Laura, who had been a normal eater until her baby's birth, became temporarily panicked by her weight gain and her increased isolation following Kimberly's birth in the dead of a New York winter. Her responses were as follows:

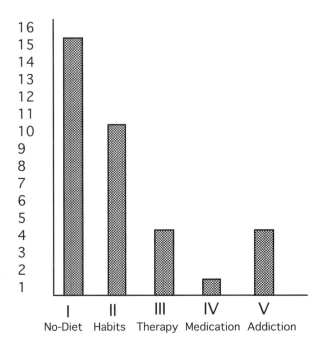

Through short-term therapy, Laura was able to reestablish her usual eating habits and curtail her tendency to undereat during the day, which led to overeating at night. Her therapy included a focus on the behavioral habit work to strengthen her commitment to eat from physical hunger. In addition, we explored Laura's anxieties about becoming a mother, and she joined a support group for new mothers in her neighborhood.

John also considered himself an alcoholic and attended Alcoholics Anonymous meetings. His mother and sister were compulsive eaters, and his father died when John was five, leaving him with deep feelings of abandonment and grief. His mother, herself depressed, died of complications from diabetes. These were John's responses:

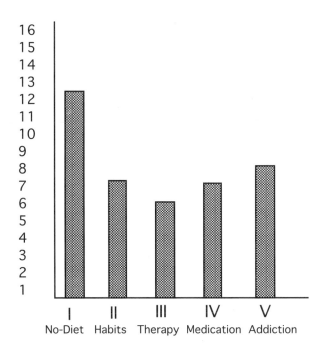

John's responses leaned heavily on both the No-Diet and the Addictions scale, but he found that by using OA to help him maintain his abstinence from sugar, he was free to eat normally and not restrict himself. Ongoing psychotherapy to resolve his issues of rage and sorrow at his parents' deaths was invaluable in helping him build a more trusting relationship with his girlfriend and to finally marry her. He was also helped by a short-term course of medication that alleviated his depression.

Your Bar Graph

Now let's look at *your* bar graph. The more your responses lean to the No-Diet and Habits approaches, the more you should concentrate on legalizing all foods and retraining your eating habits. I find this is most easily accomplished with the support of short-term therapy for eating disorders as well as the support of a behaviorally oriented eating disorder group.

The more your responses tally in the Addictions range, the more likely you will benefit from a commitment to OA. The Program suggests that newcomers immerse themselves by going to 90 meetings in 90 days. The advantage of this intensive approach is that you are quickly creating a community of support for yourself. After these three months, you can evaluate with your sponsor and your therapist whether this is truly the right approach for you.

If you scored high in Habits, you can benefit from a short-term therapy group where the emphasis is placed on correcting skewed eating patterns and distorted thinking patterns. If you measured high in the Psychotherapy section, you should consider consulting a therapist. This is particularly true if you have sexual or physical abuse in your past, unresolved grief or guilt, or if you suffer from a fear of success. The relationship with your therapist, in which you work both on your emotional struggles and your eating disorder, becomes the channel for change.

An evaluation for medication is necessary if you have suicidal feelings, ongoing depression, debilitating anxiety, chronic bulimia, or if your life is significantly damaged by your eating disorder or mood. If you answer "yes" to more than two questions, a medical evaluation is also indicated.

The poet, Walt Whitman, once said: "Do I contradict myself? I contain multitudes!" In truth, each person struggling with an eating disorder contains a variety of strengths, hopes, and experiences. It would be great if there were one easy answer for everybody, but this is not the case. Your creative integration of all these approaches will become your own personal plan of action. An individualized program will support your unique journey by respecting the complexity and richness of your human experience.

CHAPTER 12

Relapse

Quitting smoking is easy—
I've done it hundreds of times.
—Mark Twain

The Compulsive Eater's Dream: "I will become as thin as I've always wanted. I'll never binge again, and I will live happily ever after."

The Bulimic's Dream: "I will become as thin as I've always wanted. I'll never purge my food again, and I will live happily ever after."

The Anorexic's Dream: "I will never starve myself again. I will eat like a normal person, be thin, and live happily every after."

Living happily ever after—with our food and weight issues solved—is a dream fostered by diet organizations, fasting programs, health clubs, and even our own fantasies. But emotional eating problems are complicated issues which have a way of rearing their heads again and again, leading us down the path from where we came and where we vowed we would never return. The dream of living happily ever after rings hollow if we revert to our old eating patterns after resolving never to do so again.

How many times have you thought you finally made peace with your food and weight, only to find yourself going from store to store so that no one grocer will know how much junk food you were hoarding? If you are bulimic, how do you understand your return to the drive-in fast food counter at two in the morning knowing that the dumpster out back is a perfect place to purge? If you are anorexic, how do you continue to make sense of lying to your mother by telling her you just went to dinner with friends when your last meal was really two days ago?

The answer is relapse.

Relapse is a detour along the path of recovery. It occurs when we experience a breakdown in our efforts to maintain natural weight or normal eating and we slip back into old habits of bingeing, purging or starving. Once we are in the grip of relapse, we feel defeated—as if the battle were lost. We are filled with feelings of failure, hopelessness, guilt and despair. Once again we seem to be at a dead end.

The tendency to relapse is actually a normal part of healing, however, and knowing this can ease our panic and despair. In fact, we can actually view relapse in more hopeful terms—a message from our inner selves that all is not well and that something within us is still begging to be understood and addressed. Relapse is a chance to review the stress of our lives and evaluate what is not working. It provides us with another opportunity to learn and develop and grow.

In his book, *Relapse Prevention*, Dr. G. Alan Marlatt describes relapse as a fork in the road, with one path taking us in the direction of positive change and the other returning us to our familiar problems. But not every lapse must lead to relapse. When we were learning to drive a car, for example, we sometimes benefited from a mistake like overturning the wheel because it taught us new information about how to make that turn.[1] So it is with eating problems. It need not be that a lapse = relapse = collapse. We can use our lapses to lead to prolapses— sliding or falling *forward*!

Stages of Recovery

To better understand how we relapse, let's first look at the path of recovery which usually follows four stages:

In the first stage, we tend to deny we have an eating problem or that it is affecting our life. We rationalize our food problems with statements like, "I can stop compulsive eating whenever I want." "There's no connection between my emotions and bingeing." "Throwing up is okay—it helps me keep my weight down." "Plenty of people use laxatives."

When we reach the second stage, we concede that we do, indeed, have a problem. We begin to admit that the reason we feel faint while crossing the street is because we have not eaten for three days. Or a dawning humiliation sweeps over us as we pull up to a traffic light and the driver next to us stares in fascination as we wolf down ice cream, chocolate dripping down our blouse.

In the third stage of recovery, we resolve to take action to help ourselves. We join a support group or seek out therapy. We make the commitment to break our negative patterns and begin learning to live without bingeing, purging, or starving.

In the last stage of recovery, one that sustains and nourishes all we have learned, we actively pursue a satisfying and balanced lifestyle. We learn to cope with our emotions, pain, or stress without the crutch of food, and we develop a way of life which supports that commitment.

The stages of recovery from an eating problem can be compared to the ones that Dr. Elizabeth Kubler-Ross identified in her dying patients: **Denial** is the first response of the dying as it often is for the person with an eating disorder: "There must be some mistake! This can't be." This is followed by **anger**, "Why me? What did I do wrong?" Next, a **bargaining** position emerges to postpone the inevitable. The dying person may say to God, "I'll never lose my temper again, if only you let me live." The eating disorder person may say, "I promise to exercise every day if only I can lose weight." The fourth stage is **depression** accompanied by hopelessness and sadness that this problem is never going to get better. And finally, in the last stage, **acceptance**, the person stops fighting and feels a certain mixture of surrender, hope, quiet resignation, and the determination to move on.

At any point along this continuum, however, we may lose our footing, find ourselves ambushed by old habits, and begin to relapse.

Warning Signs

If forewarned is forearmed, then knowing everything we can about the signs of relapse will prepare and strengthen our coping abilities.

The most common cause of relapse is **stress**, which can come in many forms, but is most often caused by loss or change in our lives. There are permanent losses, such as the death of someone we love, an abortion, or divorce.

There are physical losses such as illness or injury or the body's decline due to aging. Financial stress, mid-life crisis, and the "empty nest" syndrome, as well as less dramatic changes, such as an argument with family or friends, moving, or sexual difficulties, can also cause stress. Actually, the very process of healing itself causes stress because we are now asking ourselves to handle life without the crutch of food.

In his book, *Love, Medicine, and Miracles*, Dr. Bernie Siegel discusses how stress connected with loss affects cancer patients. I believe his observations have significant relevance for emotional eaters: "One of the most common precursors of cancer is a traumatic loss. When a salamander loses a limb, it grows a new one. In an analogous way, when a human being suffers an emotional loss that is not properly dealt with, the body often responds by developing a new growth (cancer). It appears that if we can react to loss with *personal* growth, we can prevent growth gone wrong within us."[2]

A patient of mine, Millie, was a compulsive eater who had made great progress in coming to terms with her eating until her husband and mother died in the same year. Unable to "digest" and "metabolize" these traumatic losses, and unable to let herself fully grieve, she turned to her most trustworthy "friend" of the past—ice cream and cookies—and gained 80 pounds.

Relapse can also occur when life becomes too good, which also can feel like a stress and therefore an invitation to return to emotional eating. For this reason, even changes for the better, such as a graduation, marriage, pregnancy, new job, retirement, or vacation can provoke their own worries.

Larry returned to his old binge eating patterns while awaiting the birth of his first child. Although he was thrilled about the prospect, he was also filled with a certain dread about the new responsibilities it entailed. He feared the added financial burden the child would mean, but mostly, he feared losing his wife's exclusive attention. He turned to food to fortify himself against these mounting pressures and the uncertainties in his life over which he had no control.

There are other warning signs that should be heeded in addition to those related to loss and change. If we find ourselves coping by other excessive means, such as working too much, drinking too much, smoking, or spending too much money, we should be aware that our preoccupation with food may have found another compulsive avenue of expression. This **switching of compulsions** means that the root of our emotional eating problem remains intact even though our stress has been temporarily detoured. In this situation there is a good possibility of relapse at some point in the future.

Overeating sugar or salt-laden foods can also lead to relapse because excess sugar and salt stimulate our body's stress response by throwing its delicate chemical balance out of whack. We then crave more and more food, only to wind up feeling moody and irritable. And this irritability can again lead us to the soothing comfort of food.

Complacency is still another warning sign that relapse may be on the horizon. If life becomes too comfortable, we can slowly drift back into bingeing, purging, or starving without even realizing it. We can even be fooled into thinking that losing weight is a sign we have made peace with our emotional eating, but unless we address the issues that underlie our food problems, they will return. Carmen expressed this realization with bewilderment, as if she were the victim of a cruel hoax. "I lost 35 pounds at a diet group, and I assumed I could now eat anything I wanted because I believed I had finally solved my eating problem. And then I started bingeing again!"

Although people can fully resolve their eating problems, old patterns sometimes reappear in moments of vulnerability. **Denial** of this possibility can also set the stage for relapse. Denial means forgetting the time your boyfriend found you passed out on the bathroom floor after you had starved yourself for days. If you are bulimic, it can also mean forgetting that once you have a couple of drinks, you cannot stop bingeing and purging for the next four days.

Finally, if you are a **"Type A" personality**—as so many emotional eaters are—and you hurry through life, always rushing to reach the next goal but never letting yourself savor the process, then you are especially susceptible to relapse. "Type A" personalities often lead their lives the same way they eat—gulping rather than chewing!

Preventing Relapse

In order to discuss various strategies to help prevent relapse, we need to remember that only by getting to the underlying emotional issues which trigger eating problems is there any real hope of permanently resolving them. Without a full exploration of these deep, inner concerns, relapse is inevitable. Simply restraining ourselves from the external behavior of bingeing, purging or starving does not mean the journey is over. Full recovery is first and foremost an "inside job."

This was brought home to me in an especially poignant way by a bulimic patient of mine, Vera, who appeared for her session with a cartoon which was meaningful for her. It showed a monster lying dejectedly on a psychiatrist's couch. "I can accept I'm a monster," the monster says mournfully. "I just can't accept I'm a miserable monster."

Up to this point in her therapy, Vera had made great strides in curtailing her bingeing and vomiting, but she was still lonely, isolated, and without friends. We began to deepen our work, focusing on her early, hurtful relation-ships with her parents. She talked of her father who had sexually abused her as a child and of her mother who screamed and hit her repeatedly. These early experiences had deeply shaken her trust in all human relationships and were intimately connected with her bulimic behavior in her later life.

For us to be content with just helping her stop the bingeing and purging, would have been to put the "inner monster" of emotional eating only temporarily out of its misery. We also needed to take the misery out of the monstrous experiences Vera harbored inside. Only by uncovering those deep-seated emotions that led her to bulimia in the first place was there any real hope for full recovery or for preventing relapse in the future.

Rehearsing Situations

Many problem eaters actually have a dim, pre-conscious awareness of when their eating problems will resurface, and making this awareness conscious can help avoid a relapse.

I often ask people in my groups to imagine the next time they think they will have a problem with food. At first, everyone looks at me in amazement because they assume food problems come out of the clear blue without warning. But then someone will say, "I know! Sunday dinner at my mother's. That's usually a binge trigger for me." And another will add thoughtfully, "When Bill has to work Saturday night, I'll be all alone."

I then encourage my patients to imagine these situations ahead of time, so they can develop strategies to fortify themselves. We call this "rehearsing a relapse." The following are some sample situations for you to rehearse. What would you do in each case? I have added several possibilities, every one of which is valid. The more ways you have of intervening on your own behalf, the more prepared you will be.

Your roommate has gone away for the weekend, leaving behind her stash of ice cream and potato chips. You are lonely and bored and cannot find a "place" for yourself. Your urge to binge is mounting. How would you handle this situation?

There are several possibilities:

a. have a portion of the food and stop when you're full.

b. make a meal for yourself instead that will be nourishing and satisfying.

c. throw out the food and replace it when the urge lessens.

d. go for a walk, go to a movie, take a nap or call a friend.

e. if you do wind up bingeing, you can forgive yourself, knowing that you did the best you could in that situation and the next time is another opportunity for change.

Your boss calls you into her office and criticizes the way you handled a project. Her attitude makes you angry because you know you worked hard on it. You are afraid to express this anger to your boss and this begins to translate into a need to eat and throw up. What should you do?

You can help yourself by:

a. telling your boss that you believe you did the best you could on this project, and asking if the two of you can discuss this further. (Speaking up is one of the great antidotes to emotional eating.)

b. leaving her office and discussing with a colleague what happened and what you should do.

c. calling a friend and talking out your feelings.

d. going to the ladies room until you feel more calm, knowing that the urge to eat and throw up will pass whether or not you eat.

e. if you wind up bingeing and purging, you can forgive yourself knowing that the next time is another opportunity to help yourself.

You visit your aunt for Thanksgiving dinner. Everyone is overeating and making a joke of it. You have eaten to the bursting point when your aunt comes out with dessert: pumpkin pie, apple pie, and a chocolate cake. Your inner voice tells you that if you have dessert you are going to wind up taking laxatives. If you tell your aunt "No," she'll say, "Oh, come on. We only do this once a year." Here are some suggestions:

You can:

a. decide to have a piece of pie and let yourself enjoy some dessert without needing to punish yourself.

b. tell your family you have to stretch your legs and will be back in 20 minutes.

c. call a friend who can support you.

d. tell your aunt before dinner that you are bulimic and pressuring you to eat is like giving an alcoholic a martini.

e. if you do wind up turning to laxatives, you can forgive yourself, reminding yourself you did the best you could in that situation and the next time is another opportunity to grow.

Urge Surfing

We can also take an active approach to coping with those occasions when we get a strong urge to overeat, purge, or starve. Instead of exercising will-power or just "grinning and bearing" it, Dr. Marlatt suggests the idea of "urge surfing."[3] He compares the urge to overeat, purge, or starve to an ocean wave which starts small, builds to a crest, and then breaks and subsides. We can be swept under by the force of the wave, or we can visualize mastering the wave by climbing on the crest and riding it. This image of "riding the wave" results in a certain detachment from our eating urges so that "I'm dying for an ice cream and I have to have it" becomes "I am having an urge for ice cream even though I'm not hungry. This is a signal that something is bothering me, and I need to find another way to deal with it."

"Urge surfing" can also be an excellent meditation device. Breathe deeply and picture yourself coasting on top of the wave of emotional eating with a sense of power and triumph. Rather than giving in to your urge, just "Let It Be."

Avoiding High-Risk Situations

There comes a time in recovery when you will have to learn how to handle high-risk situations. If going to the office Christmas party with its vast array of liquor and desserts will make you vulnerable to an episode of bulimia, give yourself the permission not to go or leave before you start feeling out of control. Knowing and respecting your needs and limits will help you avoid getting into the quicksand of your eating problems.

Of course, it is not always possible to plot your life so as not to encounter difficulties, but you can plan ways to support yourself in situations over which you have no control. One of the most helpful actions to take is to call a supportive friend. Take the time to discuss what you are feeling and what you want to eat, and often you will find the intensity of the urge to eat will subside. If you cannot reach someone, choose an action incompatible with emotional eating, like going for a walk or writing in a journal.

Developing a Compassionate Attitude

Another coping skill is developing a compassionate attitude towards ourselves. The more we can see the silver lining in every cloud rather than a cloud in every silver lining, the more strengthened will be our resolve to curtail emotional eating. Caring for ourselves in spite of our human mistakes will help us view this eating journey from a calmer, more gentle perspective.

Justine had been free of anorexia for just three months when her grandmother died. In an attempt to drown her grief, Justine starved herself for three weeks before she was able to return to normal eating. She was extremely angry with herself and humiliated by what she considered a failure.

I viewed Justine's reoccurrence of anorexia very differently, though. I pointed out to her that it is common for people to have lapses during painful times. Although she had needed to "touch base" with her old security blanket of anorexia during this period of intense sorrow, her determination not to starve any more had, in fact, quickly won over. I helped her recognize that she had actually shown *strength* in resuming her commitment after three weeks, and that she could use this experience to figure out additional coping strategies for the future. What's more, her personality trait of never giving herself a break could actually *lead* her to further discouragement and problems with relapse.

In truth, the process of change is filled with fits and starts. Many of us feel like failures if we cannot sustain a heightened level of commitment at all times, or if we backslide or lose our enthusiasm. But we must learn to tolerate a certain degree of ambivalence and confusion. Compassion for ourselves is the single, most important ingredient in recovering from a relapse! After all, "Anything worth doing is worth doing imperfectly!"

Recovering from a Relapse

Let's say that it is too late for prevention techniques, and you are in the throes of relapse. What now?

1. Sit down and breathe deeply but calmly. Stay still and keep breathing.

2. Admit to yourself that your eating is out of control and is making your life unmanageable.

3. Stay calm. Let your feelings wash over you and then pass. Guilt, self-blame, and despair are normal, but they do not help anyone change. Recovery requires some amount of trial and error, and that doesn't mean making an error and then putting yourself on trial!

4. Renew your commitment to your recovery. Think back to what was working before the relapse. Remember the reasons you wanted to break free from emotional eating in the first place.

5. Decide on a plan of action. Throw away your binge foods. Write down what you will eat for today. Remove yourself from whatever situation may have provoked you.

6. Ask for help. Call a friend. Find a therapist. Join a support group. Go to an Overeaters Anonymous meeting and ask for a sponsor. If you find yourself too deeply enmeshed in your old eating patterns, consider the possibility of a medication evaluation or inpatient treatment.

7. Review the events leading up to your relapse. What were the stresses in your life? What inner thoughts and emotions, circumstances, or relationship problems could have set you off? Did you detect any other warning signals? When and where could you have intervened before the relapse escalated?

This after-the-fact evaluation will make your patterns of vulnerability clearer so you will be able to plan how to better care for yourself in the future.

Maintaining Recovery:
A Daily Plan of Action

Sustaining a daily commitment to healthy eating patterns can be fostered by keeping an eating diary. Make a copy for each day of the week:

The Daily Eating Diary

1. Did I encourage myself to eat from physical hunger?

2. Did I eat at the *first* signal of hunger, rather than letting myself get overly hungry?

3. Did I find myself eating or starving for emotional reasons today?
Boredom _____
Anger _____
Depression _____
Anxiety _____
Fatigue _____
Frustration _____
Sexual feelings _____
Transition between activities _____
Other _____

4. Which times of the day and evening were the most troublesome for me with food?

5. What alternatives did I take during those times?

6. What alternatives could I have taken?

7. What are the ways I took good care of myself today?

8. What are the ways I needed to give to myself today?

9. What emotional needs do I anticipate for tomorrow and how can I plan to take care of them?

10. Did I practice HALT (not letting myself get too Hungry, too Angry, too Lonely, or too Tired)?

11. Have I forgiven myself for any eating difficulties today, knowing I did the best I could and that tomorrow is a new day?

A Supportive Lifestyle

The final cornerstone of maintaining recovery and preventing relapse is to cultivate a supportive lifestyle.

Driven by the tyranny of the "shoulds," problem eaters tend to unwittingly increase their own stress by treating themselves as if their needs and time were unimportant. They also postpone pleasure, and this deprivation—be it of food or of emotional sustenance—leads to the backlash of overindulgence. By giving ourselves permission to rest, exercise, relax, be playful, and have satisfying compan-ionship, we are providing ourselves with the best remedy for emotional eating and the best prevention for relapse.

When I ask my patients, "What gives your life meaning besides your eating problem? What are the things that give you pleasure in life?" sometimes the answer is sor-rowfully little. I once ran a group where three women be-gan their compulsive eating when they gave up a beloved dance class because of the demands of work and family! I tell all my patients that *pleasure is preventive medicine.*

A Spiritual Connection

Many people in recovery find that developing a supportive lifestyle is connected to a spiritual awakening. A spiritual awakening means realizing you cannot solve your problems alone and that you need to find faith in something greater than yourself.

My own spiritual journey began to unfold many years ago on a visit to a small tropical island near Puerto Rico. One sunny and fragrant day, I set off on a hike down a back country road covered with a bower of leaves and vines, and lined with jasmine and mango trees. At the end of the road grew something I had never seen before—a cashew tree heavy with fruit, a paisley-shaped nut dangling from each fruit.

A small foot trail led up the side of the hill which I followed to the very top. From the hilltop I could see a breathtaking view of the ocean—aquamarine and purple—with lagoons and palm trees along the shore. I lay down on the field of soft purple grasses and breathed in the smell of the humid earth. A white heron flew overhead, with wings fluttering in the stillness. A great and warm feeling welled up in me, and I cried for the beauty, happiness, and love I felt—for life, for myself, and for all humankind.

This little corner of the world helped me realize that my connection with nature was vital to me, and each year I continued to make a pilgrimage to this hilltop. What happened in my life in New York City felt like it belonged in parentheses compared to this, and I gradually made a home for this tropical place in my heart. This experience gave a perspective to the rest of my life by reminding me that there is a larger whole than the struggles and angst of everyday life. "Those who dwell among the beauties and mysteries of the earth are never alone or weary of life."[7] I continue to actively cultivate that sense within me—an inner smile.

The serenity of my hilltop is a reflection of my spiritual self, and I can visit there whenever I want by simply knocking gently at my heart's door.

Eating problems are both similar to and different from the spiritual experience. In both, we are looking for something to take us out of ourselves, to transcend our pain. We are looking to feel whole and at peace. While an obsession with food keeps us locked in an escalating cycle of isolation and despair, a spiritual awakening opens the door to hope. It is only by cultivating a connection with ourselves and our fellow creatures that we truly embrace wholeness, that relapse is avoided and our recovery is sustained.

Questions and Answers

CHAPTER 13

Questions & Answers

1. Bingeing at Boyfriend's House

Q: I've recently started going out with someone new, and I find that whenever we spend the night together, I wind up bingeing in the middle of the night. I am ashamed that my boyfriend is going to catch me. Can you suggest anything?

A: Your saying that your boyfriend will "catch you" implies that you feel you are doing something shameful and horrible. In fact, bingeing is probably a way of taking care of yourself, of trying to nurture some of your unmet needs. Ask yourself how you are feeling before you binge. Are you scared of this new-found relationship? Are you able to express yourself sexually? Are you, like many women, embarrassed to eat a full meal in front of a new man only to wind up hungry later that night? Asking yourself these questions can help you translate what feelings the binge is trying to address.

You do not mention if bingeing or nighttime eating has always been a problem for you, or if you struggle with this more in times of stress such as when you are dating. Playing detective with yourself can help you discover specifically what is triggering you to reach for food, and then you can decide how to best intervene on your own behalf. The easiest route would be to tell your boyfriend that you enjoy a midnight snack and to prepare something for yourself ahead of time. Then you will not feel like a sneak nor be at the mercy of your impulse of the moment.

One of the most painful aspects of bingeing is the sense of shame and isolation that can sweep over you. You might want to consider joining a group for emotional eaters where the connection between overeating and relationships is addressed.

2. Weight Gain During Therapy

Q: *Two years ago I went into therapy for a number of problems. One of them was my compulsion to overeat which caused me to gain weight. Even though I feel I've made progress in other areas, I have been turning to food even more and have continued to gain weight. My therapist says I'll lose my extra weight when we better understand all my inner feelings. What do you think?*

A: People often gain weight in the course of psychotherapy because their anxiety increases when they begin working on difficult and painful issues. Food becomes a comfort to relieve this anxiety. This weight gain is usually temporary and resolves itself when the patient begins to resolve his or her problems.

However, there are cases where a bingeing problem is not given sufficient attention in therapy. Some therapists believe that insight alone will cure an eating problem and they do not discuss with their clients the nitty-gritty of what foods they eat or examine the connection between eating and emotional issues. Also, many people have an addictive relationship to food that does *not* respond to a strictly therapeutic approach which focuses solely on emotional issues. These patients need to be taught the tools and techniques for managing their compulsion. Support groups are particularly helpful in this regard.

I suggest you discuss your concerns directly with your therapist. Take more initiative to tell him or her how compulsive eating is a very real problem for you. Be candid about how unsettled you are with your weight gain and discuss with your therapist the possibility of joining an eating support group.

3. Bulimic Daughter in Therapy

Q: My daughter is eighteen and recently told us she is bulimic. My husband and I took her to a therapist, and Cathy seems to like her. But whenever I call the therapist to talk about my daughter, she says she cannot discuss her case with me. Actually, she recommends we see a therapist of our own. I'm frustrated and confused about what to do.

A: I think your daughter's therapist is right. Because of Cathy's age, she needs a therapist just for herself. One of the main issues for adolescents, and especially bulimic adolescents, is their struggle to be more separate and independent from their families. She needs to feel the therapist is her ally and not an extension of you; having a therapist of her own is a step in that direction.

If you can learn to detach from your daughter's eating problem and not get trapped in a power struggle with her, then the responsibility of resolving her bulimia will rest squarely on Cathy's shoulders. Here are some recommendations for dealing with her: Do not get into discussions with her about her eating or weight; let that be the realm of her therapy. Try not to focus your energy exclusively on Cathy and her eating problem to the exclusion of the rest of the family, and do not try to use guilt or threats to make your daughter change.

It is understandable that you are frustrated. You and your husband might consider seeing another therapist on an "as needed" basis. Support groups for parents whose child has an eating disorder could also be helpful. A hospital that has an eating disorder unit might be able to give you a referral.

4. European Vacation

Q: I am leaving on vacation soon for a two week tour of Europe. I always gain quite a bit of weight on vacation, and I'm hoping this time will be different. What can you suggest?

A: Go back and analyze what caused your weight gain on past vacations. Some common trip-ups (no pun intended) are the desire to sample all the unique and exotic cuisine of a particular country, or traveling with a tour package that provides all your meals. People on vacation often find themselves eating more than usual because they are dependent on restaurants and passively eat whatever is served. Choose a vacation package that offers sufficient opportunity to exercise and move about.

If you are traveling in a group, it can be difficult to get in touch with your own rhythm and eat consciously. Here are some suggestions: Are there times on the vacation that you might need a nap and not extra food? Each morning you might consider writing out a day's menu plan for yourself. Try providing your own breakfasts and picnic lunches in order to rely less on restaurants. Maybe you can even get a hotel room with a kitchenette.

Some people feel that vacations are the one time of year they can break out of the regular strict diet they follow at home and enjoy eating without restraint. If you are on a rigid, regimented diet in your "regular" life, your vacation may seem like the ideal opportunity to throw restriction to the wind. In that case, you will need to re-evaluate how you eat back home and find ways to make *that* more satisfying. This will make vacation food seem less like "forbidden fruit" that you cannot resist.

5. Liquid Diet

Q: My doctor recommended that I lose weight because my cholesterol level is very high. I tend to binge eat on high fat foods and cannot seem to stop. I am feeling overwhelmed and desperate and am thinking of going on a liquid diet. What is your opinion about that?

A: I can appreciate how frustrating it is to have a lot of weight to lose and want to see the quick results that a liquid diet provides. There is no doubt that liquid diets do help people lose weight. They are also appealing because they work relatively quickly and give you the illusion of being in control of your eating. What's more, the fact that many fasts are medically supervised makes them seem professional and trustworthy.

However, you need to be aware of some of the drawbacks. First of all, liquid dieting lowers your rate of metabolism and causes your body to burn calories more slowly. After the fast, when you return to normal eating again, you will gain weight more quickly than usual because your metabolism is still lowered. The panic at seeing weight come back so easily often causes people to eat even more because they feel they have lost control of their bodies.

A second drawback to liquid diets is that the deprivation involved can backfire, causing people to make it up to themselves by overeating at a later date. Excessive restriction always has this rebound effect.

The most glaring drawback to liquid diets is that they do not help you examine the problems, situations, or habits that may be causing you to overeat. Liquid diets may help you avoid eating, but they do not teach you how to deal with food cravings or handle the emotions and stresses that cause you to binge eat. Just as you cannot learn to play tennis by swimming, you cannot learn to deal with your eating problems by fasting.

A more reasonable solution is to find a structured and moderate food plan which you can live with comfortably, and introduce an exercise program into your life to help you reach a natural, healthy weight *permanently.* Many people often find the support of a group to be extremely helpful and comforting. Be sure to find a group that helps you cope with both your eating behavior and the emotional stresses in your life.

6. Daughter Denies Anorexia

Q: My daughter has begun exercising and working out during her spare time. She has lost a lot of weight and looks very thin, but it seems she is never able to sit still for a minute. I told her she shouldn't lose any more weight and should cut back on her working out. She told me that I just don't understand, that she has hit on a good way to lose weight. What do you think?

A: There is enormous pressure on women, especially young women, to be trim. Sometimes teenagers get involved with fads, go overboard for awhile and then return to moderation. However, exercise can become compulsive for many young women, a way to "undo" the excesses of overeating. This is called "exercise bulimia."

You need to determine if your daughter falls into the exercise bulimia category: How much of her school life or social life is being damaged by her preoccupation with working out? Does she feel guilty after eating or overly anxious when she cannot exercise? Has she reduced her socializing with friends and replaced it with exercise? Does her conversation focus on weight, diet, and food, to the exclusion of other topics? Do you feel that what really motivates her is not so much the enjoyment of moving her body but her fear about gaining weight?

If this is so, you need to confront her with your belief that she is exercising to deal with her anxiety about her body. Try to help her plan a moderate food and exercise program. If she needs additional help, suggest a professional consultation with a therapist or nutritionist who specializes in eating problems.

7. Summer Embarrassment

Q: It's summer again and I'm still fat. I get so angry at myself that I had all winter to do something about my weight and didn't. Now with the warm weather here, I'm still too self-conscious to go the beach or really enjoy myself. Do you have any ideas about what I can do in the meantime?

A: There is no "meantime." As the saying goes: "Life is not a dress rehearsal. We only have the present and it is now!" Whether you are fat or thin, this is the only life you have and it is meant to be lived fully, regardless of your size. It is true that large people tend to be more self-con-scious and self-critical because our society is prejudiced against large bodies, especially women's bodies. But what really stands out in your question is your feelings of not deserving pleasure.

Millions of people believe that their life's problems would be solved if only they lost weight. The truth is that preoccupation with weight can often serve as a smoke screen for deep inner feelings of not being entitled to pleasure. I suggest you try to determine whether there are reasons, other than your weight, that might make you feel undeserving of an enjoyable summer. Are you struggling with something that is causing you to feel anger or guilt? These are the two areas that give people the most trouble in feeling entitled to happiness.

Now consider the following idea: If you were never going to lose weight for the rest of your life, would you continue to put your life on hold or would you try to do the best you can with who you are now? Can you, right now, give yourself some of the things you fantasize having at a slimmer weight? Working to identify and resolve your personal barriers to deserving happiness will help you get free from the *inside*. This will lead to your becoming the person you want to be regardless of your size!

8. Husband Has Gained Weight

Q: My husband has gained an enormous amount of weight since we've been married and is probably now over 300 pounds. Sometimes it feels like he is going to eat us out of house and home. He absolutely refuses to go for counseling despite my pleading. At this point I'm feeling so angry and hurt that I don't know what to do.

A: It is understandable that you should feel angry and hurt because your husband is out of control, and you are powerless to stop him. As with other addictions, compulsive eating becomes a family problem causing those involved with the overeater to worry and suffer. You probably feel that if your husband really cared enough about you, he would stop or go for help. But when people are in the throes of an addiction, they are powerless. What's more, your pleading with him to stop can contribute to a cycle of bitterness and resentment between the two of you. This may cause him to further overeat to spite you for trying to control him.

To break the cycle, you need to extricate yourself. Tell your husband of your concerns, but then separate from his problem. I recommend you go to a family support group, O-Anon meeting (a branch of Overeaters Anonymous just for families of emotional eaters), or an Al Anon meeting (although this program is designed for families of alcoholics, many issues are similar). The support you will get at these meetings will help you learn what you can and cannot do to assist you husband. You will hear the message that we are all essentially powerless to change other people and that we can only change ourselves. You will also learn how to keep the focus on you and not make his weight your life's work.

9. Switching Compulsions

Q: I've been feeling more in control with overeating, but lately I've been shopping a lot more and spending money like it's going out of style. What's going on?

A: The name of the game you describe is "switching compulsions"—exchanging one method of easing tension for another. People who eat or drink excessively, gamble, or engage in compulsive sex are usually avoiding facing their fears, loneliness, anger, or pain. Any compulsive activity is like a mood altering drug which serves to anesthetize you to whatever life problems you are having trouble confronting. Compulsive people crave intensity and enjoy bouncing from emotional highs to lows. Moderation feels boring.

To let go of a compulsion, try letting yourself sit and just "be" without excess food or excess spending and get to know what the inner you is really craving. When you do this, you might experience a deep sadness or emptiness, a feeling of void, or nothingness. Try to translate what this means. Are you depressed? Are there memories within you that are too hard to face? Do you feel a lack of meaning in your life or a lack of close connection with people?

A combination of physical exercise and a program of meditation seems to work best for people who are trying not to switch compulsions. Joining a self-help group where other people are working on similar issues in their recovery can also be helpful.

10. Anorexic Daughter in Denial

Q: My daughter is anorexic but refuses to change. She even admits she is often dizzy and hungry. Why won't she give it up?

A: Even though your daughter admits to discomfort, the "benefits" of anorexia are greater for her at this time. Actually, anorexics are usually in denial about how hungry, cold, or scared they really are. Instead, they report positive feelings about not eating, such as "I finally feel in charge of my life," "I'm more organized than ever," or "I'm working more efficiently now." The underlying feeling is that they have everything under control.

People with anorexia try to trade in their many doubts, fears, and uncertainties about themselves for one manageable problem—starvation. While they may feel helpless about their feelings and the course of their lives, the triumph and power of overriding their hunger more than compensates. What's more, in the beginning stage of starvation, people also experience a euphoria which they are loathe to give up. This euphoria has a physiological basis akin to the "runner's high."

I suggest you share this information with your daughter and tell her you understand what she is going through. There are many support groups for anorexics and their families. Your daughter needs a chance to be with other girls like herself and break through the isolation that usually surrounds this illness. The fact is that anorexia *is* an illness and it requires treatment. Parents should not take "no" for an answer from their child who needs help.

11. Home for the Holidays

Q: I'm going home for the holidays and I always have trouble with food when I'm with my family. Then I wind up hating myself. What can you suggest?

A: Your problem is shared by many adult children. One of my clients described that whenever she returned home to visit her parents, her first stop was always to check out the refrigerator. Going home can bring up feelings of being young and vulnerable. Family reunions can stir up power struggles about eating and not eating which are replays of old conflicts between dependence and independence.

Here are some suggestions: When you are back home, try to stay in touch with your own grownup needs, be they for space, privacy, or the amount of food you want. Then, try to stay firm about holding onto these needs and boundaries. Do not let yourself be coerced into eating more than you want. Hold onto your adult self, even if it means bringing work with you, making phone calls to friends, going out for a walk. And remember, each time you go home, you will be able to use it as a learning experience for the next time around.

12. Wife with an Eating Disorder

Q: My wife recently told me she has a bingeing problem and has asked me to help her. But whenever I make a suggestion, she blows up and tells me to leave her alone. Now what?

A: You must really feel in a bind. Your wife asks for your help on one hand, then slaps you down. People with eating problems often seem like victims one minute and victimizers the next. Although your wife may appreciate giving you the responsibility for her eating at first, she then begins to resent that you are in the controlling and superior position.

Maintain a stance of neutrality. This is necessary for your well-being as well as hers. Do not become enmeshed in your wife's problem because this will make it easier for her to blame *you* than to look at her own inner distress. Al Anon, the support group for spouses of alcoholics, has recommended that spouses learn to "detach with love." In other words, you can be supportive and concerned, but leave the problem squarely on your wife's shoulders.

You *can* ask her how she would specifically like you to help, but do not let her manipulate you into being her policeman or conscience. Do not let your relationship revolve around her eating problem, but continue to pursue the areas of enjoyment that you both share, as well as pursuing your own interests. Also, let your wife know, verbally and physically, your honest interest in and affection for her regardless of her problem with food.

13. Power Struggle with Mother

Q: My mother has been trying to get me to lose weight all of my life by criticizing and hassling me about what I eat. Now that I'm older I find that every time I try to stop bingeing, I wind up sabotaging myself because I just don't want to give my mother the satisfaction of giving her what she wants. I really need help with this because I want to learn to feel more in control of my eating just for myself. What do you recommend?

A: It is wonderful that you have made the connection between your difficulty giving yourself permission to eat healthily and your inner feeling of wanting to spite your mother. This need to get back at her is obviously keeping you stuck.

I once had a patient whose mother badgered her constantly to become a doctor. Even though this young woman really wanted to go to medical school, her mother's forcing it down her throat made it seem like the last thing in the world she wanted to do. As we worked together, we discovered that her mother's repeatedly telling her what profession to choose was a way of dominating and trying to control her daughter. Probably, if her daughter finally did get her M.D., her mother would regret losing this power to keep telling her what to do!

What I am suggesting to you by this story is that your mother's need to control you has given her a certain power in your life and you are resentful of this. What was once a battle between you and your mother over your losing weight has now become a battle within yourself.

There are four steps you can take to set in motion the process of resolving this issue. First, write a detailed history of all the memories and incidents from your childhood which illustrate your mother's controlling and hurtful behavior about your weight. Be as specific as possible in order to re-experience your feelings. You need to re-experience these emotions because the anger and hurt trapped inside of you are the cause of your self-sabotage.

The next step is to read what you have written to a trusted friend or a therapist. Don't be afraid to cry or get angry or let your feelings come up. Having another person witness your pain and anger is a healing experience. Then, write a letter to your mother (this is for your benefit and therefore need not be mailed) in which you tell her how she has interfered with your ability to regulate your weight. The goal of this exercise is to help you externalize your pent-up feelings.

The last step in this process is for you to decide whether or not *you* want to lose weight. Accepting yourself just as you are can be a powerful gift to yourself. If you do decide on weight loss, focus on a small and do-able goal. For example, increase your amount of exercise or eat less fatty foods.

14. Laxatives

Q: I worry about my weight and I use laxatives a lot. I heard on a talk show that people can get addicted to using them. How do I figure out if I am headed in that direction?

A: First of all, let's look at the facts. Laxatives DO NOT result in weight loss because the calories from the foods you eat are already absorbed in your system by the time the laxatives go to work. Laxatives stimulate the colon to produce a bowel movement, and this is too late in the digestive process to avoid calorie absorption. The only reason people feel thinner after they use laxatives is because of the water loss, but this dehydration is only temporary.

You do not mention how many laxatives you use. Occasional use will not lead to addiction, but excessive use will impair the function of your colon. The colon is a muscle that gets exercised through the natural digestive processes, but by overriding that natural process, laxatives make your body progressively dependent on them in order to function.

Take this problem seriously and work on breaking the cycle. Here are three ways to do that. First, detoxify slowly from laxatives. It is best to do this under medical supervision since the colon needs to slowly regain its strength. Secondly, you need to recognize and repeat to yourself that laxatives absolutely *do not* cause weight loss. Instead of solving problems, they cause extra problems.

The third area to explore is the emotional meaning that taking laxatives has for you. Some people are driven to use laxatives because they feel cleansed and purged of whatever "crappy" feelings they are unable to "digest." What feelings are you trying to purge that may be uncomfortable? Why have you come to mistrust your natural body functions? How can you support yourself in a healthy way with your eating?

15. Husband's Help Backfires

Q: I desperately want to lose weight and my husband wants that too. We decided he would help me, but since then everything has backfired. I wind up cheating behind his back and feeling very guilty. I'm afraid to tell him that his pressure is making me worse because he'll accuse me of not really wanting to lose weight. I'm in a dilemma, and I wonder if you can help me.

A: Of course you are in a dilemma. Any time we make someone else responsible for our behavior, it is a sure set-up for failure. Your situation reminds me of a 15-year-old bulimic patient who asked her mother to lock up the refrigerator at night. Guess what this girl did after her mother went to sleep? She would begin "The Hunt for the Hidden Key."

Your husband has become your policeman and you have become the criminal. You need to take back the power you gave him and monitor your own self. Then you need to ask yourself whether your weight loss endeavor is for him or for you. We all want to look and feel our best, but you seem to be expressing some panic beyond that natural wish. You speak of "desperately" wanting to lose weight, and I wonder why you are so desperate. Has your weight become an issue in your relationship? Often one spouse's complaints about the other's weight is a smoke screen for something deeper which is more difficult to express. If you need some extra support, join a group where everyone is committed to working on their eating problems and helping one another.

16. *Thanksgiving Dinner for Relatives*

Q: I am making Thanksgiving dinner for my family this year, but I'm worried about how to handle the food. I'm on a food plan and would like to just serve what I can eat so I won't be tempted. On the other hand, I want to prepare a traditional meal with all the trimmings for my family, but I'm scared I'll go out of control with all that food. What do you suggest?

A: The key ingredient is not to set yourself up to feel deprived by creating "your" food vs. "their" food. Forbidden fruit is always the sweetest! I believe you should make a meal that makes *you* feel comfortable.

You should be prepared for guests who bring a contribution—a pie, a bottle of wine. Rehearse how you would handle this. Will you binge on the pies, wolfing them down after the company has gone, or make some peace ahead of time by allowing yourself to eat everything moderately? Perhaps it would help to make a commitment to a friend or someone at your party about what and how much you plan to eat so you do not feel so overwhelmed by the temptations of the moment. Even if you do have trouble, though, you can return to healthy eating the very next day. Put your difficult eating episode behind you and make sure you do not try to play "catch up" by limiting your next day's food to compensate. This will only perpetuate the cycle of problem eating.

17. Bulimic Daughter Refuses Help

Q: *My daughter is bulimic and refuses to go for help. My husband, son, and I are quite concerned because she seems to be eating and purging more and more. She also has been drinking too much. We feel helpless. How and where can we get help?*

A: Your daughter may be suffering from two addictions, alcoholism and food addiction. In addition, your family is suffering from having to live with her addictions. The term "co-dependence" has been coined to describe how family members become trapped in the disease of the person they love.

Often families do not seek help because they believe that nothing will change until the addicted person is willing to go for counseling. However, when a loved one is struggling with an addictive disease, family members do need to get help for themselves. A growing body of evidence shows that the addicted person often seeks help *only after* the family has taken the necessary first steps towards therapy. Treatment centers and self-help groups for family members have become increasingly available in recent years.

Many bulimics are addicted both to alcohol and to bulimia. Both of these addictions are progressive and can be life-threatening. When your daughter eventually enters treatment, the therapist can judge which is more advanced, and the treatment can be prioritized accordingly.

One approach which is effective in getting resistant patients to seek help is called family intervention. This is a process where your family meets with a therapist, without your daughter present, and discusses how her alcoholism and bulimia are affecting each of you. Together you will plan how to best confront your daughter in a gentle but firm way. She will then be asked to attend one or more family sessions where, in a loving context, she will be faced with the fact that her disease is affecting the entire family.

If your daughter refuses to attend, the family can still be helped by continuing to meet together. If your daughter is financially dependent, do not be afraid to use that leverage to get her to enter treatment. Bulimia and alcoholism are serious addictions and must be treated as such.

18. Feeling Fat after Weight Loss

Q: Recently I've lost a lot of weight, but still feel fat. Even though my friends tell me how great I look, it doesn't make a dent. Why is this? What can I do?

A: We all carry around in our minds a mental image of how we look which has developed from all the years of living with ourselves, looking at our bodies, and the feedback we get from other people. When our physical appearance changes, as it does when we lose weight, our minds experience a delay in registering this new image. This is similar to the phantom limb syndrome in which a person continues to feel the existence of an arm or leg even though they have lost it.

Although the psychological awareness of weight loss is slower to register than the physical weight loss itself, there are certain steps you can take to help you integrate your new body image. Buy clothes that fit your current size; this will help you adjust your perception of your body's new boundaries. Look at yourself in a full length mirror and trace your contour with chalk. Observe your chalk image over the next two weeks and try to view it objectively in order to comprehend that this is the real you. Ask yourself whether you have any emotional investment in continuing to see yourself heavier than you really are. Many women feel their fat serves as a protection, especially in their relationships with men. And many people use "feeling fat" as an excuse not to do new things in their life that are scary, such as look for a better job.

You also mention that your friends have been complimenting you. How does that feel for you? Do you worry that they might be jealous and not like you as much anymore? Many women fear weight loss because of competitive feelings that get stirred up with their friends. Feeling heavier than you really are could be your way of trying to protect yourself from having to face the possibility of your friends' envy.

You may need help deciphering the meaning of your "fat feelings." Joining a group of women who are working of body image issues may be a way to get the support and feedback you need.

19. Preventing Baby's Weight Problem

Q: I have had a food problem all my life. Now I'm pregnant and am wondering if there is anything I can do so my baby will not have to suffer the way I did.

A: Mother Nature gives babies a perfectly adapted mechanism which regulates when they are hungry and when they are full. You can foster this in-born mechanism by feeding your baby on demand. If you follow your baby's cues, he will tell you when to feed him and when to stop. As your child grows, he will continue to need the autonomy to state when, what, and how much food he wants, and you will need to respond to his cues.

The surest way to start a food problem with a child is to become involved in power struggles about eating. Avoid using food as a reward or punishment, or criticizing or teasing a child about their eating habits.

You might also want to investigate those factors in your background that contributed to your eating problem. The more specific and conscious you become, the more you will avoid making the same mistakes with your child. I often hear patients discuss how their parents were anxious that their children not grow up fat. But in conveying so much anxiety, the parent perpetuated in the child the idea that food is dangerous and appetite scary.

We should also acknowledge that increasing evidence points to the role of genetics in determining weight, and that as a parent you are powerless to control heredity. Also, children learn by example, so the more you can free yourself from your own difficulty with food, the better perspective your child will have on the role of food in his life!

20. Summer Vacation with Friends

Q: I live alone, and for the most part, I am able to struc-ture my food comfortably for myself. This summer I'm go-ing to be sharing a house with a group of women friends, and I'm getting scared at how easily I can get out of control with my eating, particularly when there is a lot of party-type food around. Do you have any recommendations?

A: If you are accustomed to a more controlled way of eating, it can feel overwhelming to be bombarded by choices and temptations. I suggest that each day you try to organize your foods, especially those that tend to give you trouble. For example, one day you might plan to have something sweet without guilt. On another day, you can decide to have a glass of wine. Try to match the food you eat with what you are really hungry for.

Also, rather than depriving yourself of what everyone else is eating (which sooner or later can backfire into a binge), give yourself a portion. The best way to do this is in a buddy system. Team up with another woman in the house who also has food fears and talk to her on a daily basis about how you want to handle eating. Finding someone in the house should not be too difficult, since most women, sadly enough, will tell you within the first half hour of meeting how fat they feel and how much weight they want to lose. Other options for teaming up might be to find a buddy back home and calling him or her daily from your summer house. You could also join a support group such as Overeaters Anonymous. Don't forget that your vacation is about relaxing and enjoying yourself, not obsessing about food!

21. Am I a Compulsive Eater?

Q: I have often heard the expression "compulsive eater." I'm trying to figure out if that's me. What's the difference between a compulsive eater and someone who just eats a lot?

A: A world of difference! Some people will go to a party and eat too much because the food is delicious. The next day they will return to eating "normally"—eating when they are hungry and stopping when they are full. These same people might also go on vacation, sample everything from soup to nuts, gain ten pounds, come home and then take off the weight without undue stress.

Compulsive eaters, on the other hand, go to a party, overeat whether or not the food is delicious, and then feel so guilty that the next day they keep on eating! Compulsive eaters go on vacation, gain ten pounds, come home and eat more because they feel so discouraged about their weight gain. Compulsive eaters cannot stop because they are emotionally driven to the food and constantly preoccupied by it. They have no willpower because the eating takes on a life of its own and is not under their control.

How do you know which you are? If you make a sincere attempt to stop eating compulsively and begin a process of trying to tune in to eating when you are hungry and stopping when you are full, you can probably train yourself to respond to your inner cues. Then you are probably not a compulsive overeater. Remember that learning new eating behaviors is a process, so give yourself time and support to work this out. However, if you notice that your overeating is progressing and beginning to interfere with your work, social life, or self esteem, you are probably a compulsive eater, and you should seek help.

22. Fear of Weight Gain During Pregnancy

Q: I'm pregnant and I'm worried about all the weight I'm going to gain. I don't want this to interfere with enjoying my pregnancy, but I can't stand the idea of getting fat. Help!

A: Ironically, when people feel fat, they get discouraged and eat more. Since pregnant women tend to feel powerless over their growing bodies, they often resign themselves to overeating with impunity. It is important that you tell yourself repeatedly throughout your pregnancy that your body is growing bigger because of a new baby. The growing fetus and increases in body fluids and blood volume do cause weight gain. This is usually shed about six weeks after delivery. The American College of Obstetricians and Gynecologists recommends a weight gain of 20 to 30 pounds during pregnancy.

Try to follow these rules of thumb: Eat when you are hungry and stop when you are full, and try to separate your emotional stress from your physical hunger. Fluctuating shifts in hormones, in your blood sugar level, in your moods, and water retention all contribute to the increased appetite that many pregnant women report. Think about joining an exercise group for pregnant women—the exercise will also help raise your blood sugar and stave off hunger.

Also, I think you might want to investigate why the idea of getting fat is so scary for you. Many women do retain some of their pregnancy weight even after the baby is born. What's more, it is not unusual for people to gain weight as they get older. Decoding the meaning of your fear of fat will help you accept your body no matter what its age or weight.

23. Quitting Smoking

Q: I really would like to give up smoking but I'm afraid of gaining weight if I do. What can you suggest?

A: People often turn to smoking for the same reason they turn to food. It relieves and soothes tension, it distracts us, it keeps us company. Tobacco smoking is a very real addiction and it is very easy to substitute one addiction for another.

You can also develop a love affair with food after you quit smoking in order to counter the symptoms of withdrawal from nicotine, which include nervousness, irritability, difficulty sleeping, depression, and anger. Keep in mind that these symptoms will pass with time whether or not you eat over them.

Choose a time in your life to stop smoking when you are relatively free from external pressure. Quitting when you are under great stress, such as when your work responsibilities are more intense, will set you up for failure. Also, try to alter your routine in order to break the habits you associate with smoking. When you begin to crave a cigarette or food do not just sit there passively and wait for the urge to pass, but substitute another action to absorb your attention. For instance, instead of a cigarette with your morning coffee, take a walk. The more variety of activities you can provide for yourself, the more tools you then have to combat the cravings.

There is evidence that nicotine raises the rate of your metabolism. Exercise does the same thing. Substituting an exercise regime for smoking will help you avoid weight gain when you quit smoking.

24. Night Time Bingeing

Q: I live alone and wake up at night and find myself bingeing. I don't binge during the day, but at night I'm up several times, visiting my refrigerator. What can I do?

A: First of all, it is important to determine whether you are eating enough food during the day, especially at your evening meal. If you delay eating long enough, you may not even be aware of how hungry you are until it is time to go to sleep, and your body reasserts its needs. It is important, therefore, to eat sufficiently during the day so hunger does not creep up on you in the evening.

You might plan to have a satisfying snack right before you go to bed. A warm glass of milk contains tryptophan which promotes sleep. Also, you could prepare something ahead of time for when you wake up, so you are not at the mercy of your food cravings when you're only half awake. You might even want to keep that prepared food by your bed, so you can eat it when you wake up without getting out of bed. This might help you fall back to sleep more quickly as well.

When you speak of "visiting" the refrigerator, it sounds like you are lonely and looking for company in food. You remind me of the line in the old country and western song, "Looking for Love in All the Wrong Places." You might consider finding yourself a warm and cuddly stuffed animal instead. Don't laugh—it works!

25. Confused by Diet Organization

Q: Two years ago my sister and I went to a diet organization because we both wanted to lose some weight. I followed their food plan and lost weight but then started bingeing. From then on I've been either bingeing or dieting and gaining or losing up to fifteen pounds a month. Can you make any suggestions to help me get out of this cycle? I'm desperate.

A: It seems that by going on that diet two years ago you have tampered with your body's mechanism of regulating hunger and fullness, and this has thrown you into a vicious cycle of bingeing and dieting. Although you say that you wanted to lose weight, it very well may be that the weight at which you started out was ideal for you because you had no bingeing problems at that time.

To break out of this cycle, you need to stop dieting. This idea probably frightens you because you think you might just continue to overeat and gain weight. However, the truth is that your dieting is fueling your binges by setting up a deprivation state of "famine" relieved only by "feasting." Eat whatever you want when you are hungry and you will see that your bingeing will ebb.

You may also find that when you *stop* dieting you will lose weight because the binge/diet cycle interferes with your metabolism's efficiency. You may naturally settle at your weight of two years ago. Then you have two choices—living at that weight and making peace with it or increasing your exercise dramatically.

26. High Blood Pressure and Doctor's Reaction

Q: *I have high blood pressure and my family doctor gave me a diet to follow to lose weight. I haven't been able to follow it very well, though, and when I saw him last time he scolded me and told me not to come back if I didn't start losing weight. What do I do now?*

A: I cannot tell you how many times people have told me that their doctors threatened them to either lose weight or to not come back. It seems as though doctors believe that people can and will change if they are threatened. The truth is that this rarely works. I think his scolding you is a way of avoiding the fact that he doesn't really know how to help you.

The most effective way to help someone like you, who needs to lose weight for medical reasons, is to work with a team of professionals. This means a coordinated effort by a nutritionist, a therapist to discuss any emotional problems that stand in your way, and a medical doctor. It is important for you to realize you are not a failure in your weight loss endeavor, but that you need more supportive help. It may be necessary for you to switch to a doctor who has more awareness of eating problems.

27. Returning Home Following Weight Gain

Q: I am going back home to my family for my summer vacation (they live out of state), and I've gained 30 pounds since the last time I've seen these relatives. I'm embarrassed and ashamed to have them see me this way, and I am even thinking of not going. Can you help me out?

A: You need to ask yourself the following question: If you don't go home, will you wind up feeling angry at yourself or will you feel you have done something truly nurturing and protective? My sense is that it could be important for you to go home despite the shame you are feeling. This does not mean it will be easy or painless, but it may give you an opportunity to see if you can treat yourself compassionately under difficult circumstances.

The worst scenario is that you go home and everyone will have a critical comment about your weight. In that case it would be helpful to be prepared with a stock answer such as, "Yes, I have gained weight lately. Anyway, I'm glad to be home. How have you been?" The important thing is not to apologize. If you don't make a big deal about it, no one else will either. If you become apologetic, you will inadvertently be inviting criticism.

The most probable scenario, however, is that your family will notice your weight gain, wonder why, and then move on to a different topic. You are assuming your family is going to be as negative about your weight gain as you are. Try to remember you are more than just your weight. People love you for many reasons, and your size is just one aspect of you (and it is neither good nor bad).

Also, remember that the reason you are going home is to enjoy and connect with your family. Plan ahead of time what would maximize your pleasure in the visit—would it be spending some time alone each day? Having a private conversation with your most favorite relative? Keeping in touch with friends back home? Going for walks? Bringing an absorbing book you've been wanting to read? Once you are back home, think about becoming part of a group to help you work on issues of compulsive eating and self-esteem.

28. Non-Compliant Mother with Diabetes

Q: I don't know whether this is really an eating disorder question or not, but I am very worried about my mother. She was recently diagnosed with diabetes and was given a diet to follow by her doctor. She has been unable to follow it and has even gained some weight lately. My mother is a smart woman but doesn't seem to want to help herself. I'm afraid for her. What should I do?

A: Because it is so painful to watch someone we love hurt themselves, we have a tendency to rush in and try to rescue. Invariably, this causes power struggles and bitterness. I am assuming, by the way, that your mother has all her faculties and is not suffering from a depression that would need special psychological intervention.

Ultimately, your mother is responsible for taking care of her own health, although there are a number of things you might do to help. Try to get her to talk about her feelings. Is she denying her diagnosis? Is she angry at her body for "betraying" her? Is she feeling defiant? All of these are common reactions to the news that we have an illness, but sometimes just being able to identify the feelings can be helpful in stopping self-destructive behavior.

You do not mention whether your mother had problems with eating before her diabetes was diagnosed, in which case she may need therapy or a support group for compulsive eaters. I also recommend a consultation with a nutritionist and a diabetic support group, where she will be able to share with others and get the encouragement she needs. The local diabetes association in your town will be able to provide referrals for such a group.

29. Life Changes: Mother's Death and a Divorce

Q: My mother died two months ago, and I am totally out of control with my eating. I'm bingeing all the time and can't seem to stop. Can you suggest something?

Q: Six months ago my husband and I got divorced. Since then I've put on 50 pounds and have been overeating tremendously. The decision to divorce was mutual, so I cannot blame him. I guess it hasn't been so easy for me. I need to get back on track. Help!

A: Both of you are dealing with feelings of loss and have turned to overeating to help you. Food is the most legal and most available mood altering drug around. Both of you are using food to numb or comfort or distract yourselves. It is probably easier for you to focus on the problem of overeating than your feelings of helplessness, anger, despair, loneliness, or guilt that these losses may have stirred up.

Loss also brings up feelings of mourning, and I believe that when mourning or grief gets "stuck," food problems move in. Both of you need to face the full range of emotions you have about these losses. You should be talking with friends or family about your experiences and letting yourselves cry. (Often emotional eaters feel uncomfortably out of control with tears and use food to stuff them down).

When are your most vulnerable times with food? At night? On weekends? During those times, you need to plan some people-oriented strategies instead. Emotional eaters often isolate themselves and short-circuit their needs by turning to food rather than calling on the support of others. If this is the case, short term therapy can be helpful. Isolating with pastry needs to be replaced by intimacy with people!

30. Exercise Inertia

Q: I really want to start exercising but cannot get myself motivated. What should I do?

A: Exercise can be a wonderful way for you to feel in partnership with your body, that the two of you are allies. Let's try to first understand what your inertia means. What fears are holding you back from committing to the exercise you say you want? How do you imagine yourself once you are more fit? Is there something about that image that worries you? What are the payoffs in keeping yourself stuck? Sometimes, when people begin to exercise, they get more in touch with their bodies and feel a surge of sexual or aggressive feelings which scares them. "Flexing one's muscles" also has the connotation of empowering yourself. Is there something that would be frightening about that?

Secondly, try to discover ways of changing your "stuck" behavior regardless of the emotional inhibitions which hold you back. Choose an activity that is "you" and that is realistic for your energy level. If your expectations are greater than what you can sustain, you will be setting yourself up for defeat. Even if you start out with just extra walking, you are doing something more than you did yesterday. Your goal should be progress not perfection. Making a plan to exercise with a friend is a tried and true technique.

With all the exaggerated and destructive emphasis in the media for women to look like pumping iron champions, it may take courage to just accept yourself with the body you own. Can you allow your body to feel valid and attractive just as it is right now? That is another legitimate alternative!

Conclusion

Once we declare peace with emotional eating, the search for meaning and wholeness in our lives still continues. Compulsive eating, chronic dieting, bulimia, and anorexia were our attempt to feel whole and cohesive. Now we need to turn toward life and relationships to help us connect in a deeper way with the inner source of our vitality.

This prayer captures the essence of that quest:

> "Let us treasure the time we have, and resolve to use it well, counting each moment precious—a chance to apprehend some truth, to experience some beauty, to conquer some evil, to relieve some suffering, to love and be loved, to achieve something of lasting worth. 'Alas for those who cannot sing, but die with all their music in them.' "

> May we "fulfill the promise that is in each of us, and so to conduct ourselves that, generations hence, it will be true to say of us: The world is better because, for a brief space, they lived in it."[1]

When we work towards declaring peace with emotional eating, we give ourselves the opportunity to live and express all the rich and varied music that is within us. Here's to life! Good luck!

FOOTNOTES

INTRODUCTION

1. Weldon, Fay. "Is Thin Better?" *Allure* magazine. New York: June 1994.

CHAPTER 1: THE FEAR OF FAT

1. Hill, Carol. *Jeremiah 8:20*. New York: Random House, 1970.
2. Chernin, Kim. *The Obsession*. New York: Harper & Row, 1981.
3. Canetti, Elias. *Crowds and Power*. New York: Continuum, 1971.

CHAPTER 2: SHAME

1. Kaufman, Gershen. *Shame: The Power of Caring*. Rochester, VT: Schenkman Books, 1985.
2. Gravitz, H. & Bowden, J. *Recovery: A Guide for Adult Children of Alcoholics*. New York: Simon & Schuster, 1987.
3. Alice Miller, quoted by John Bradshaw in *Healing the Shame that Binds You*. Deerfield Beach, FL: Health Communications, 1988.
4. Whitfield, Charles. *Healing the Child Within*. Deerfield Beach, FL: Health Communications, 1987.

CHAPTER 3. SEXUALITY AND SELF EXPRESSION

1. Offit, Avodah. *Night Thoughts: Reflections of a Sex Therapist*. New York: Congdon and Lattes, 1981.
2. Hite, Shere. The Hite Report. New York: Dell, 1981.
3. Sherfey, Dr. Mary Jane. *The Nature and Evolution of Female Sexuality*. New York: Vintage Books, 1973.

CHAPTER 4. ANGER AND ASSERTIVENESS

1. Thanks to Vince Gerardi for this insight.
2. Woititz, Janet. *Struggle for Intimacy*. Deerfield Beach, FL: Health Communications, 1985.
3. Garner, David, M.D. and Bemis, Kelly, PhD. "Cognitive Therapy for Anorexia Nervosa," p. 135 in *Handbook of Psychotherapy for Anorexia Nervosa & Bulimia*, edited by D. Garner and P. Garfinkel. New York: The Guilford Press, 1985.

4. Lerner, Harriet Goldhor, PhD. *The Dance of Anger.* New York: Harper and Row, 1989.
5. Kernberg, Otto. "Love, the Couple and the Group: A Psychoanalytic Frame," *The Psychoanalytic Quarterly*, Vol. 49, No. 1.

CHAPTER 5: OVERCOMING THE FEAR OF SUCCESS

1. Bruch, Hilde. *Eating Disorders*. New York: Basic Books, 1973.
2. Hollis, Judi, Ph.D. *Fat is a Family Affair.* Center City, MN: Hazelden, 1985.
3. Eichenbaum, Luise & Orbach, Susie. *Between Women.* New York: Penguin Books, 1987.
4. Thanks to Carol Gladstone, ACSW, for this turn of phrase.
5. Viorst, Judith. *Necessary Losses.* New York: Simon & Schuster, 1986.
6. Warner, Samuel. *Self-Realization and Self-Defeat.* New York: Grove Press, 1966.
7. Strean, Herb. *Why People Fail.* New York: Wynwood Press, 1992.
8. Rubin, Theodore Isaac, M.D. *Compassion and Self-Hate.* New York: Ballantine Books, 1975.

CHAPTER 6: ADDICTION

1. *Alcoholics Anonymous.* New York: Alcoholics Anonymous World Services, 1976.
2. *Ibid.*
3. Bill B. *Compulsive Overeater*. Minnesota: CompCare, 1981.
4. *Alcoholics Anonymous, op. cit.* p. 83.
5. *Alcoholics Anonymous, op. cit.* p. 88.
6. Hollis, Judi, Ph.D. *Fat is a Family Affair.* Center City, MN: Hazelden, 1985.

CHAPTER 7: NO MORE DIETS, DEPRIVATION

1. Special thanks to Susie Orbach, Geneen Roth, Carol Munter, and Jane Hirschmann for pioneering the no-diet/no-deprivation path.
2. Tenzer, Susan. "Fat Acceptance Therapy: A Non-Dieting Group Approach to Physical Wellness, Insight and Self-Acceptance," in *Overcoming Fear of Fat.*, edited by Drs. Laura Brown & Esther Rothblum. New York: Harrington Park Press, 1989.
3. An outgrowth of this approach of trusting and honoring our hunger is the Fat Acceptance movement. Despite our culture's relentless pursuit of thinness, there is a growing feminist movement addressing fat oppression and offering fat acceptance therapy. Organizations such as The National Association to Aid Fat Americans champion the rights of fat people in employment, health care, and most of all in self-love.

CHAPTER 8: HABITS

1. Milne, A.A. *When We Were Very Young*. New York: E.P. Dutton, 1924.
2. Bryan, Nancy Ph.D. *Thin is a State of Mind*. Minneapolis, MN: CompCare, 1980. p. 28.

CHAPTER 9: PSYCHOTHERAPY

1. Folk song: Simon and Garfunkel.
2. Hollis, Judi, Ph.D. *Fat is a Family Affair*. Center City, MN: Hazelden, 1985.
3. I am indebted to Craig Johnson for the formulation of some of these questions in *The Handbook of Psychotherapy of Anorexia and Bulimia*. Editors D. Garner & P. Garfinkel. New York: Guilford, 1985.
4. The groups I lead are for compulsive eaters and bulimics. Until starvation is under control, an anorexic's ability to relate to others is sorely diminished, and the focus needs to be individual psychotherapy.
5. Thanks to Andrea Schneer, CSW, friend and colleague, for this insight.
6. Shakespeare, William. *Macbeth*. Act 4, Scene 3.

CHAPTER 10: MEDICATION, MOOD, MALLOMARS

1. I am indebted to Dr. Barry Rand, attending psychiatrist at Maimonides Medical Center, Brooklyn, New York, for his generosity in stimulating many of the ideas contained in this chapter.
2. The American Psychiatric Association. *A Quick Reference to the Diagnostic Criteria from DSM-IV*. Washington, D.C. 1994. p. 252.
3. *Ibid*. p. 254.
4. *op cit*. p. 251.
5. Kaye, W. & Weltzin, T. "Neurochemistry of Bulimia Nervosa" in *The Journal of Clinical Psychiatry*. Vol. 52, October 1991 supplement. p. 22.
6. "Practice Guidelines for Eating Disorders" in American Psychiatric Association Practice Guidelines of *The American Journal of Psychiatry* 150:2 February, 1993. Washington, D.C., p. 213.
7. The American Psychiatric Association. *A Quick Reference to the Diagnostic Criteria from DSM-IV*. p. 161-162
8. Klein, D. M.D. & Wender, P. M.D. *Understanding Depression*. New York: Oxford University Press, 1993.
9. Drs. J. Mitchell, S. Specker & M. de Zwaan. "Comorbidity and Medical Complications of Bulimia Nervosa" in *J. of Clinical Psychiatry* 52:10, Oct 1991, p 15.
10 Gise, Dr. Leslie. "Premenstrual Syndrome: Which Treatments Help?" in *Medical Aspects of Human Sexuality*. February, 1991. p. 12.
11. Dr. Leslie Gise. Personal Communication.
12. Klein & Wender. *op. cit.* p. 111.

13. Drs. P. Garfinkel & D. Garner. "Use of Tricyclic Antidepressants in Anorexia Nervosa and Bulimia Nervosa" in *The Role of Drug Treatments for Eating Disorders*. Brunner/Mazel. New York, 1987. p. 53.

CHAPTER 11: HOW TO PLAN YOUR OWN PATH

1. Sheppard, Kay. *Food Addiction*. Deerfield Beach, FL: Health Communications, 1989.

2. Roth, Geneen. *Breaking Free from Compulsive Eating*. New York: Bobbs Merrill, 1984.

3. Virtue, Doreen. *The Yo-Yo Syndrome Diet*. New York: Harper & Row, 1989.

4. Bilich, Marion, Ph.D. *Weight Loss from the Inside Out*. New York: Seabury Press, 1983.

5. Hollis, Judi, Ph.D. *Fat is a Family Affair*. Center City, MN: Hazelden, 1985.

6. Hirschmann,J. & Munter, C. *Overcoming Overeating*. New York: Addison-Wesley, 1988.

CHAPTER 12. RELAPSE

1. Marlatt, G. Alan. *Relapse Prevention - Maintenance Strategies in the Treatment of Addictive Behaviors*. New York: The Guilford Press, 1985.

2. Siegel, Bernie, M.D. *Love, Medicine, and Miracles*. New York: Harper Collins, 1986.

3. Marlatt, G. Alan. *op.cit.*

4. A quote by Rachel Carson.

CONCLUSION

1. Stern, Chaim, Editor. *The New Union Prayer Book for the Days of Awe*. New York: Central Conference of American Rabbis, 1979.

About the Author

Mary Anne Cohen, C.S.W., B.C.D. is a professional psychotherapist and director of The New York Center for Eating Disorders. She has hosted a New York radio show on eating disorders, *French Toast for Breakfast,* and has authored a series of internationally popular self-help tapes on resolving eating problems.

Ms. Cohen has also appeared on national television and lectured extensively to professional and community groups. She is a member of the American Anorexia and Bulimia Association, and is on the Board of Directors of The Eating Disorder Council of Long Island.

Ms. Cohen maintains a private practice in Brooklyn, NY and supervises and teaches other professionals.

Outside of office hours, she can be found hiking down back country roads or dancing the mambo.

Mary Anne Cohen, C.S.W., B.C.D.
The New York Center for Eating Disorders
490 Third Street
Brooklyn, New York 11215
(718) 788-6986

ORDER FORM

French Toast for Breakfast is available at bookstores and libraries. Copies may also be ordered from Gürze Books.

FREE Catalogue
The Gürze Eating Disorders Bookshelf Catalogue has more than 80 books, tapes, and videos on eating disorders and related topics, including body image, self-esteem, feminist issues, and more. It is a valuable resource that includes listings of non-profit associations and facts about bulimia, anorexia nervosa, and binge eating. This catalogue is handed out to individuals and family members by therapists, educators, and other health care professionals throughout the world.

Please send me:

____ **FREE** copies of the *Gürze Eating Disorders Bookshelf Catalogue*

____ copies of *French Toast for Breakfast*
    $12.95 each (1-4 copies)
    plus $1.95 per copy for shipping and handling

____ copies of *French Toast for Breakfast*
    $10.95 each (5+ copies)
    plus $1.55 per copy for shipping and handling

NAME _____

ADDRESS _____

CITY, ST, ZIP _____

PHONE _____

Mail a copy of this order form to:

Gürze Books (FTB)
P.O. Box 2238
Carlsbad, CA 92018

Phone orders accepted:
(800) 756-7533